# Fatty Liver Diet Cookbook

Eat Right and Live Bright with 2000 Days of Liver-Loving Recipes for Lasting Vitality. Includes a 30-Day Meal Plan

*Audrie Scott*

# Table of Contents

# THE LIVER: YOUR BODY'S SILENT WORKHORSE

The liver, often described as the body's silent workhorse, is indispensable in maintaining our overall health and vitality. Nestled beneath the ribcage on the right side of the abdomen, this remarkable organ quietly carries out many essential functions while remaining unassuming and modest in its demeanor. From detoxifying the blood to metabolizing nutrients, storing energy, and producing vital proteins, the liver's tireless efforts are awe-inspiring.

In the **"Fatty Liver Diet Cookbook"** pages, we embark on a culinary journey that celebrates the liver's unsung heroism, exploring an array of delectable recipes designed to nourish and support this indispensable organ while tantalizing your taste buds. Through the harmonious blend of nutrition and flavor, we seek to provide a unique culinary experience that pays homage to the liver and fosters a deeper understanding of its significance in maintaining our well-being. Join us in unlocking the culinary secrets that empower the liver, ensuring it continues to perform its invaluable tasks with grace and resilience.

# 1. INTRODUCTION

## 1.1   THE GROWING CONCERN: RISE OF FATTY LIVER DISEASE GLOBALLY

A growing concern has cast a shadow over the global healthcare landscape in recent years: the relentless rise of fatty liver disease. This insidious condition, characterized by fat accumulation in the liver cells, has silently surged into one of the most prevalent liver disorders worldwide. It knows no borders, affecting individuals across diverse ages, ethnicities, and socioeconomic backgrounds. While obesity and excessive alcohol consumption have historically been recognized as primary risk factors, the emergence of non-alcoholic fatty liver disease (NAFLD) has added complexity to this health crisis. NAFLD, often associated with sedentary lifestyles and unhealthy dietary choices, has become a major driver behind the alarming surge in liver-related issues. From Asia to the Americas and everywhere in between, healthcare professionals and researchers are grappling with the formidable challenge of addressing this epidemic, underscoring the urgent need for heightened awareness, early detection, and lifestyle interventions to stem the tide of fatty liver disease.

The implications of this global health crisis are far-reaching. If not properly managed, fatty liver disease has the potential to advance into more serious stages such as non-alcoholic steatohepatitis (NASH) and cirrhosis, leading to liver failure and transplantation. Moreover, the comorbidities associated with fatty liver disease, including diabetes and cardiovascular issues, compound the already substantial burden on healthcare systems worldwide. As healthcare providers and policymakers grapple with this burgeoning crisis, there is a pressing need for comprehensive strategies that address the root causes of fatty liver disease, from promoting healthier lifestyles to advancing medical research and therapeutic interventions. In an age where prevention is often hailed as the best medicine, the global rise of fatty liver disease serves as a stark reminder that proactive measures are essential to safeguard the liver health of generations to come.

## 1.2  THE LIFELINE OF YOUR BODY: UNDERSTANDING THE LIVER'S FUNCTIONS

First and foremost, the liver is a detoxification powerhouse. It filters and cleanses the blood, removing harmful substances, toxins, and waste products that can accumulate due to our everyday activities and environmental exposures. This detoxification process is a cornerstone of the liver's role in maintaining our overall health, ensuring that the blood coursing through our veins remains free of potentially harmful compounds. Additionally, the liver metabolizes various nutrients, including Carbs, proteins, and fats, ensuring that they are efficiently utilized by the body or stored for future energy needs. Furthermore, the liver synthesizes essential proteins, such as albumin and clotting factors, vital for blood clotting and maintaining fluid balance. Through its multifaceted functions, the liver truly emerges as a silent yet indispensable guardian of our well-being, deserving our admiration and care.

## 1.3  THE CRUCIAL ROLE OF DIET IN LIVER HEALTH

Diet plays a pivotal role in maintaining optimal liver health, serving as a powerful tool in preventing and managing liver conditions. What we consume profoundly impacts the liver's functions as it processes the nutrients, fats, and toxins that enter our bodies. A diet that maintains a balance and includes ample fruits, vegetables, lean proteins, and whole grains can supply the vital nutrients and antioxidants necessary to aid the liver's detoxification mechanisms and decrease the potential for fat accumulation in this organ. On the contrary, overindulging in sugary, high-fat, and processed foods can place undue stress on the liver, increasing the risk of developing non-alcoholic fatty liver disease (NAFLD). Hence, dietary choices serve as a cornerstone for nurturing a healthy liver and preventing the onset of liver diseases, underscoring the critical link between what we eat and the well-being of this vital organ.

# 2. PART I: COMPREHENSIVE UNDERSTANDING OF FATTY LIVER

## 2.1  FATTY LIVER DISEASE: TYPES AND DIFFERENCES

### 2.1.1  Causes and Risk Factors:

The onset and progression of fatty liver disease are influenced by a complex interplay of causes and risk factors that underscore its multifaceted nature. While the exact etiology remains a subject of ongoing research, certain factors have been identified as key contributors to the development of this prevalent health concern. Excessive consumption of high-calorie, processed foods laden with unhealthy fats and sugars is a leading cause, as it can overwhelm the liver's capacity to metabolize fats, accumulating triglycerides within liver cells. Sedentary lifestyles and obesity also heighten the risk, amplifying the strain on the liver and promoting fat storage within the organ. Insulin resistance, often associated with conditions like metabolic syndrome and diabetes, can further exacerbate fatty liver disease by disrupting the delicate balance of glucose and fat metabolism. Additionally, genetics can play a role, with some individuals being more predisposed to developing the condition. Alcohol abuse remains a well-recognized risk factor, though it is essential to distinguish between alcoholic and non-alcoholic fatty liver disease, as both can have distinct causes and consequences. These causes and risk factors collectively highlight the need for a multifaceted approach to prevent and manage fatty liver disease, ranging from dietary modifications and physical activity to addressing underlying health conditions.

### 2.2.1 Recognizing Symptoms: Early and Advanced Stages:

It is vital to acknowledge the symptoms of fatty liver disease for timely intervention and effective management, as the condition can progress through distinct stages. In its early stages, fatty liver disease often presents with subtle or nonspecific symptoms, making it challenging to diagnose. Individuals may experience fatigue, mild abdominal discomfort, and a general sense of malaise. As the disease advances, more noticeable symptoms may manifest, including persistent abdominal pain, unintended weight loss, and an enlarged liver that can be identified through a physical checkup. Additionally, Jaundice, characterized by the skin and eyes turning yellow, can occur in more severe cases, indicating potential liver damage. However, it's important to note that many people with fatty liver disease may remain asymptomatic, underscoring the importance of regular medical check-ups and screening for those at risk. Early detection and lifestyle modifications can significantly improve outcomes and prevent the progression of fatty liver disease to more severe stages, such as non-alcoholic steatohepatitis (NASH) or cirrhosis.

### 2.3.1 Potential Complications and Long-Term Impacts:

Fatty liver disease, if left unchecked, can lead to a cascade of potential complications and long-term impacts on one's health. As the condition progresses, it may evolve into non-alcoholic steatohepatitis (NASH), characterized by liver inflammation and damage. NASH, on the other hand, can develop into cirrhosis, a condition characterized by the replacement of liver tissue with scar tissue, leading to a decline in liver function. Cirrhosis raises the risk of liver failure and increases susceptibility to liver cancer, making early intervention crucial. Beyond liver-related issues, fatty liver disease has systemic consequences, increasing the risk of cardiovascular problems, diabetes, and metabolic syndrome. It underscores the significance of addressing the condition proactively through lifestyle changes and regular medical monitoring to mitigate its potential long-term impact on overall health.

# 3. PART II: THE SCIENCE OF NUTRITION AND LIVER HEALTH

## 3.1 HOW DIET INFLUENCES LIVER FUNCTION

### 3.1.1 The Metabolic Connection:

Fatty Liver and Metabolic Syndrome: The link between fatty liver disease and metabolic syndrome is complex and multifaceted, with both conditions often occurring in tandem and influencing each other. Metabolic syndrome encompasses increased blood sugar levels, irregular lipid profiles, hypertension, and abdominal obesity as interconnected risk factors. These factors elevate the risk of experiencing cardiovascular disease, diabetes, and other health complications.

Fatty liver disease, specifically non-alcoholic fatty liver disease (NAFLD), frequently coexists with metabolic syndrome. These conditions often share common factors like insulin resistance and obesity. Insulin resistance, a key characteristic of metabolic syndrome, can result in the pancreas producing excess insulin. This surplus insulin can lead to the accumulation of fat Within the liver, thus aiding in the development of NAFLD. Conversely, having NAFLD can worsen insulin resistance, creating a harmful cycle that exacerbates metabolic syndrome. This intricate connection between fatty liver disease and metabolic syndrome emphasizes the importance of comprehensive management and lifestyle interventions. Simultaneously addressing both conditions through methods like weight management, consistent physical activity and adopting a well-rounded diet can substantially lower the likelihood of complications and enhance overall health. Early detection and intervention are also essential. People with metabolic syndrome should be screened for NAFLD, and vice versa, to effectively manage these intertwined health challenges.

### 3.2.1 Micronutrients Essential for Liver Health:

Micronutrients play a pivotal role in supporting and maintaining liver health, serving as essential components in the intricate metabolic processes and detoxification functions carried out by this vital organ. Among the micronutrients crucial for liver health, some of the key players include:

1. Vitamin E: This powerful antioxidant helps protect liver cells from oxidative damage and inflammation, two factors closely associated with liver disease. It also aids in preventing the progression of fatty liver disease.
2. Vitamin C: Another antioxidant, vitamin C, supports the liver by reducing oxidative stress and promoting the synthesis of important liver detoxification enzymes. It can also aid in the regeneration of liver tissue.
3. Vitamin B group: The B vitamins, especially folate, B12, and B6, are essential for various metabolic processes within the liver. They help convert food into energy, support DNA repair, and synthesize important molecules like glutathione, a key antioxidant.
4. Vitamin D: Emerging research suggests that vitamin D may have a role in protecting against Liver conditions, which encompass non-alcoholic fatty liver disease (NAFLD), along with other diseases. It is involved in immune system regulation and inflammation control.
5. Selenium: This trace element is a component of several enzymes that help the liver detoxify harmful substances and protect against oxidative damage.
6. Zinc: Zinc is essential for the metabolism of Carbs, fats, and proteins, which are processes that heavily involve the liver. It also plays a role in wound healing and immune function, indirectly benefiting liver health.
7. Iron: Iron is vital for various liver functions, including producing hemoglobin and storing iron reserves. However, excessive iron can be harmful, so maintaining a balance is crucial.
8. Copper: Copper is involved in forming enzymes that help metabolize iron, and it plays a role in the transport of bilirubin, a waste product processed by the liver.

Achieving a balanced and nutritious diet by incorporating a variety of lean proteins, whole grains, fruits, vegetables, and nuts into your meals can provide the necessary micronutrients to support liver health.

However, consulting with a healthcare provider or nutritionist before taking supplements is essential, as excessive intake of certain micronutrients can harm the liver and overall health.

### 3.3.1  The Detoxification Process: How the Liver Cleanses Your Body:

The liver serves as the body's chief detoxification center, pivotal in the intricate process of cleansing and purifying the bloodstream from harmful substances and waste products. This detoxification process is a complex and highly coordinated series of biochemical reactions carried out by liver cells, known as hepatocytes, and involves several distinct phases.

- **Phase 1**: In this initial phase, the liver enzymes work to transform fat-soluble toxins and chemicals into water-soluble compounds, making them more amenable to elimination from the body. This transformation process often involves oxidation, reduction, and hydrolysis reactions, which prepare the toxins for further processing in phase 2.

- **Phase 2:** Here, the liver conjugates the water-soluble toxins produced in phase 1 with specific molecules, such as glutathione, sulfate, or amino acids. This conjugation makes toxins less toxic and more easily excretable through urine or bile. This phase involves various enzymes and pathways, including the cytochrome P450 system.

- **Phase 3**: After phase 2, the now conjugated toxins are transported into the bile or released into the bloodstream for excretion. Those destined for elimination through malice eventually enter the intestines, excreted from the body through feces. Those passed through the bloodstream are filtered by the kidneys and expelled through urine.

The liver's detoxification prowess is not limited to processing external toxins; it also handles endogenous waste products, such as bilirubin (a derivative of red blood cell breakdown) and ammonia (a byproduct of protein metabolism). These waste products are efficiently converted and excreted, preventing their buildup to harmful levels in the bloodstream.

Moreover, the liver plays a vital role in metabolizing drugs, hormones, and other substances the body needs for daily functioning. This ensures these compounds are processed and eliminated efficiently, maintaining overall physiological balance. While the liver is remarkably resilient and efficient in its detoxification functions, it is important to support its health through a balanced diet, hydration, and a lifestyle that minimizes exposure to harmful substances. Understanding and appreciating the liver's role in detoxification underscores the importance of maintaining its health for the body's overall well-being.

# 4. BREAKFAST RECIPES
## 4.1  PAPAYA BOWL

| PREPARATION TIME | COOKING TIME | SERVING |
|---|---|---|
| 10 mins | 0 mins | 1 |

**INGREDIENTS**
1 cups papaya, chunks
½ banana
½ cup plain Greek yogurt
½ tsp lime zest
1 tbsp honey

**DIRECTIONS**
1. Slice a banana, chop some papaya, and set it aside for topping.
2. Blend papaya chunks, half a banana, plain Greek yogurt, and lime zest until you have a smooth mixture. Add honey according to your preference.
3. Put smoothie mixture in a Bowl and add toppings
4. Smoothie bowl is ready to serve

**Nutritional facts /value (per serving)**

| Cal: 260 | Carbs: 38g | Protein: 11g | Total Fats: 2g | Sodium: 40mg |
|---|---|---|---|---|
| Pott: 840mg | Calcium: 160mg | Phos: 140mg | Fiber: 4g | Sugar: 26g |

## 4.2  DETOX BOWL

| PREPARATION TIME | COOKING TIME | SERVING |
|---|---|---|
| 10 mins | 0 mins | 1 |

**INGREDIENTS**
1 cup spinach or kale
½ cucumber sliced
½ avocado
Juice of ½ lemon
1 small green apple, sliced
½ cup unsweetened almond milk
1 tsp chia seeds (optional)

**DIRECTIONS**
1. Steam the spinach and let it cool.
2. Add steamed spinach, cucumber, avocado, apple, lemon juice and almond milk in a blender and blend until mixture becomes smooth. Add chia seeds if you prefer
3. Put the smoothie mixture in a bowl and it is ready to serve.

**Nutritional facts /value (per serving)**

| Cal: 280 | Carbs: 31g | Protein: 6g | Total Fats: 18g | Sodium: 160mg |
|---|---|---|---|---|
| Pott: 900mg | Calcium: 140mg | Phos: 150mg | Fiber: 13g | Sugar: 14g |

## 4.3    TURMERIC AND MANGO SMOOTHIE

| PREPARATION TIME | COOKING TIME | SERVING |
|---|---|---|
| 10 mins | 0 mins | 1 |

**INGREDIENTS**
1 cup mango, chunks
½ banana
½ tsp turmeric powder
½ tsp freshly grated ginger
½ cup coconut milk
1 tbsp honey (optional)

**DIRECTIONS**
1.  add the mango chunks, half banana, turmeric powder, freshly grated ginger, and coconut milk in a blender. Blend them until becomes a smooth mixture
2.  If you like sweet taste, add 1 tsp of honey.
3.  Put the mixture in a serving bowl and serve cold.

**Nutritional facts /value (per serving)**

| Cal: 320 | Carbs: 63g | Protein: 4g | Total Fats: 8g | Sodium: 10mg |
|---|---|---|---|---|
| Pott: 740mg | Calcium: 45mg | Phos: 75mg | Fiber: 6g | Sugar: 48g |

## 4.4    WALNUT AND BLUEBERRIES BOWL

| PREPARATION TIME | COOKING TIME | SERVING |
|---|---|---|
| 10 mins | 0 mins | 1 |

**INGREDIENTS**
1 cup blueberries
¼ cup walnuts
½ cup Greek yogurt
½ tsp cinnamon
1 tbsp honey

**DIRECTIONS**
1.  Add blueberries, walnuts, yogurt and cinnamon in a blender and blend it until it becomes a smooth mixture.
2.  If you like sweet taste add 1 tsp of honey.
3.  Put the mixture in a serving bowl and serve cold.

**Nutritional facts /value (per serving)**

| Cal: 380 | Carbs: 40g | Protein: 13g | Total Fats: 21g | Sodium: 60mg |
|---|---|---|---|---|
| Pott: 380mg | Calcium: 180mg | Phos: 220mg | Fiber: 6g | Sugar: 28g |

## 4.5 CARROT AND GINGER SMOOTHIE

| PREPARATION TIME | COOKING TIME | SERVING |
|---|---|---|
| 10 mins | 0 mins | 1 |

| INGREDIENTS | DIRECTIONS |
|---|---|
| 1 large carrot, chopped<br>½ banana<br>½ tsp freshly grated ginger<br>½ cup almond milk, unsweetened<br>1 tbsp flax seeds | 1. Peel and chop the carrot. Blend chopped carrot, banana, ginger, almond milk and flax seeds together to make a smooth mixture<br>2. Put smoothie mixture in a bowl and add toppings of your choice like kiwi chunks<br>3. Smoothie bowl is ready to serve. |

**Nutritional facts /value (per serving)**

| Cal: 250 | Carbs:43 | Protein: 6g | Total Fats: 9g | Sodium: 160mg |
|---|---|---|---|---|
| Pott: 750mg | Calcium: 220mg | Phos: 140mg | Fiber: 11g | Sugar: 21g |

## 4.6 BEETROOT AND BERRY SMOOTHIE

| PREPARATION TIME | COOKING TIME | SERVING |
|---|---|---|
| 10 mins | 0 mins | 1 |

| INGREDIENTS | DIRECTIONS |
|---|---|
| 1 small beetroot, cooked, peeled, and cubed<br>1 cup mixed berries (strawberries, blueberries, raspberries)<br>½ banana<br>½ cup Greek yogurt<br>1 tbsp honey (optional) | 1. Add all the ingredients in a blender and blend them until a smooth mixture is formed.<br>2. Put smoothie mixture in a bowl and add sliced strawberry as topping if you like.<br>3. Smoothie bowl is ready to serve. |

**Nutritional facts /value (per serving)**

| Cal: 280 | Carbs:60 | Protein: 10g | Total Fats: 2g | Sodium: 150mg |
|---|---|---|---|---|
| Pott: 660mg | Calcium: 200mg | Phos: 210mg | Fiber: 10g | Sugar: 40g |

## 4.7   BANANA AND WALNUT OATMEAL

| PREPARATION TIME | COOKING TIME | SERVING |
|---|---|---|
| 5 mins | 10 mins | 1 |

### INGREDIENTS
½ cup rolled oats
1 cup almond milk, Unsweetened
1 ripe banana, mashed
¼ cup walnuts, chopped
½ tsp cinnamon
1 tbsp honey (optional)

### DIRECTIONS
1. Add oats and almond milk in a saucepan and boil it then let it cook for 5 minutes. Add mashed banana, chopped walnuts and cinnamon.
2. Cook for 2 more minutes
3. Add honey if you like your oatmeal sweet.

**Nutritional facts /value (per serving)**

| Cal: 400 | Carbs:60 | Protein: 10g | Total Fats: 15g | Sodium: 160mg |
|---|---|---|---|---|
| Pott: 530mg | Calcium: 120mg | Phos: 220mg | Fiber: 7g | Sugar: 17g |

## 4.8   ALMOND AND BLUEBERRY OATMEAL

| PREPARATION TIME | COOKING TIME | SERVING |
|---|---|---|
| 5 mins | 10 mins | 1 |

### INGREDIENTS
½ cup rolled oats
1 cup almond milk, unsweetened
½ cup fresh blueberries
1 tbsp almond butter
1 tsp honey (optional)
¼ tsp almond extract (optional)

### DIRECTIONS
1. Add oats and almond milk in a saucepan and boil it then let it cook for 5 minutes. Add almond butter and blueberries in it.
2. Cook for 2 more minutes
3. Add honey and almond extract if you like your oatmeal sweet.

**Nutritional facts /value (per serving)**

| Cal: 350 | Carbs:52 | Protein: 9g | Total Fats: 12g | Sodium: 160mg |
|---|---|---|---|---|
| Pott: 310mg | Calcium: 280mg | Phos: 170mg | Fiber: 8g | Sugar: 11g |

## 4.9   APPLE AND CINNAMON OATMEAL

| PREPARATION TIME | COOKING TIME | SERVING |
|---|---|---|
| 5 mins | 10 mins | 1 |

| INGREDIENTS | DIRECTIONS |
|---|---|
| ½ cup rolled oats<br>1 cup almond milk, unsweetened<br>1 small apple, diced<br>½ tsp cinnamon<br>1 tbsp almonds, chopped<br>1 tsp honey (optional) | 1.  Add oats and almond milk in a saucepan and boil it then let it cook for 5 minutes. Add diced apple, chopped almonds and cinnamon.<br>2.  Cook for 2 more minutes<br>3.  Add honey if you prefer sweet taste. |

**Nutritional facts /value (per serving)**

| Cal: 350 | Carbs:56g | Protein: 9g | Total Fats: 10g | Sodium: 160mg |
|---|---|---|---|---|
| Pott: 350mg | Calcium: 200mg | Phos: 200mg | Fiber: 8g | Sugar: 19g |

## 4.10   MIXED BERRIES OATMEAL WITH CHIA SEEDS

| PREPARATION TIME | COOKING TIME | SERVING |
|---|---|---|
| 5 mins | 10 mins | 1 |

| INGREDIENTS | DIRECTIONS |
|---|---|
| ½ cup rolled oats<br>1 cup unsweetened almond milk<br>½ cup berries (strawberries, blueberries, raspberries)<br>1 tbsp chia seeds<br>1 tsp honey (optional) | 1.  Add oats and almond milk in a saucepan and boil it then let it cook for 5 minutes. Add berries and chia seed.<br>2.  Cook for 2 more minutes<br>3.  Add honey if you prefer sweet taste. |

**Nutritional facts /value (per serving)**

| Cal: 330 | Carbs:54g | Protein: 9g | Total Fats: 9g | Sodium: 160mg |
|---|---|---|---|---|
| Pott: 320mg | Calcium: 220mg | Phos: 220mg | Fiber: 11g | Sugar: 14g |

## 4.11 SPINACH AND MUSHROOM OATMEAL

| PREPARATION TIME | COOKING TIME | SERVING |
|---|---|---|
| 5 mins | 15 mins | 1 |

### INGREDIENTS

½ cup rolled oats
1 cup water or vegetable broth
1 cup fresh spinach, chopped
½ cup mushrooms, sliced
1 clove garlic, minced
½ tsp olive oil
Salt to taste
Pepper to taste
1 tbsp Parmesan cheese, grated (optional)

### DIRECTIONS

1. Begin by selecting a saucepan and placing it over a medium flame. Heat up a dash of olive oil. Toss in the mushrooms and minced garlic, allowing them to sauté for approximately 4 to 5 minutes.

2. Introduce the chopped spinach into the pan and continue to cook for an additional 2 minutes.

3. Now, add the rolled oats and vegetable broth to the mixture, bringing it to a gentle boil. Allow this delightful blend to simmer for an additional 5 minutes, allowing the flavors to meld.

4. To season your dish, add a pinch of salt and a dash of pepper to suit your personal taste preferences. Serve this nourishing creation piping hot.

### Nutritional facts /value (per serving)

| Cal: 250 | Carbs:40g | Protein: 12g | Total Fats: 5g | Sodium: 400mg |
|---|---|---|---|---|
| Pott: 560mg | Calcium: 150mg | Phos: 240mg | Fiber: 8g | Sugar: 12g |

## 4.12 PUMPKIN PIE OATMEAL

| PREPARATION TIME | COOKING TIME | SERVING |
|---|---|---|
| 5 mins | 10 mins | 1 |

### INGREDIENTS

½ cup rolled oats
1 cup almond milk, unsweetened
¼ cup pumpkin puree, canned
½ tsp pumpkin pie spice (or a mixture of cinnamon, nutmeg, and cloves)
1 tbsp pecans, chopped
1 tsp honey(optional)

### DIRECTIONS

1. Add oats and almond milk in a saucepan and boil it, then let it cook for 5 minutes. Add pumpkin puree and pumpkin spices

2. Cook for two more minutes.

3. Add honey if you prefer a sweet taste.

### Nutritional facts /value (per serving)

| Cal: 320 | Carbs:50g | Protein: 10g | Total Fats: 160g | Sodium: 320mg |
|---|---|---|---|---|
| Pott: 320mg | Calcium: 200mg | Phos: 220mg | Fiber: 8g | Sugar: 6g |

## 4.13  BANANA WALNUT PANCAKE

| PREPARATION TIME | COOKING TIME | SERVING |
|---|---|---|
| 10 mins | 15 mins | 2 |

### INGREDIENTS

1 cup whole wheat flour
1 ripe banana, mashed
¼ cup walnuts, chopped
1 tsp baking powder
½ tsp cinnamon
1 cup almond milk, unsweetened
1 egg
1 tbsp honey (optional)

### DIRECTIONS

1. Combine all the dry components in a mixing bowl. In a separate bowl, whisk together almond milk, an egg, and honey until thoroughly blended.

2. Incorporate the wet ingredients into the dry mixture, ensuring a well-mixed batter.

3. Grease a nonstick skillet with a touch of oil and place it over medium heat.

4. To create the pancakes, ladle approximately 1/4 cup of batter onto the heated griddle. Cook until you observe surface bubbles forming, then flip and continue cooking until both sides achieve a delightful golden-brown hue.

5. Your delectable pancakes are now ready to be served

**Nutritional facts /value (per serving)**

| | | | | |
|---|---|---|---|---|
| **Cal:** 280 | **Carbs:** 47g | **Protein:** 9g | **Total Fats:** 8g | **Sodium:** 260mg |
| **Pott:** 410mg | **Calcium:** 150mg | **Phos:** 160mg | **Fiber:** 6g | **Sugar:** 13g |

## 4.14  BLUEBERRY AND ALMOND PANCAKES

| PREPARATION TIME | COOKING TIME | SERVING |
|---|---|---|
| 10 mins | 15 mins | 2 |

### INGREDIENTS

1 cup whole wheat flour
¼ cup almond meal
1 tsp baking powder
½ tsp cinnamon
1 cup almond milk, unsweetened
1 egg
1 cup blueberries, fresh or frozen
1 tsp honey (optional)

### DIRECTIONS

1. Combine all the dry components within a bowl, thoroughly mixing them.

2. In a separate bowl, blend almond milk, an egg, and honey until they are well combined.

3. Mix both the mixtures, ensuring a thorough incorporation, and gently fold in the blueberries.

4. Grease a nonstick skillet with a small amount of oil and place it over medium heat.

5. To create your pancakes, ladle approximately 1/4 cup portions of the batter onto the heated griddle. Cook until you notice bubbles forming on the surface, then flip and continue cooking until both sides attain a delightful golden brown color.

**Nutritional facts /value (per serving)**

| Cal: 320 | Carbs: 54g | Protein: 12g | Total Fats: 9g | Sodium: 160mg |
|---|---|---|---|---|
| Pott: 360mg | Calcium: 200mg | Phos: 200mg | Fiber: 8g | Sugar: 11g |

## 4.15  CINNAMON APPLE PANCAKES

| PREPARATION TIME | COOKING TIME | SERVING |
|---|---|---|
| 10 mins | 15 mins | 2 |

| INGREDIENTS | DIRECTIONS |
|---|---|
| 1 cup whole wheat flour<br>½ tsp baking powder<br>½ tsp cinnamon<br>½ cup applesauce, unsweetened<br>½ cup almond milk, unsweetened<br>1 egg<br>1 small apple, finely grated<br>1 tsp honey (optional) | 1. Begin by thoroughly combining all the dry ingredients in a mixing bowl.<br>2. In a separate bowl, whisk together almond milk, an egg, applesauce, grated apple, and honey until they are well incorporated.<br>3. Merge the wet ingredients into the dry mixture, ensuring a thorough blend.<br>4. Grease a nonstick skillet with a small amount of oil and place it over medium heat.<br>5. To create your pancakes, pour approximately 1/4 cup portions of the batter onto the heated griddle.<br>6. Cook until you observe bubbles forming on the surface, then flip and continue cooking until both sides attain a delightful golden brown color. |

**Nutritional facts /value (per serving)**

| Cal: 240 | Carbs: 50g | Protein: 8g | Total Fats: 3g | Sodium: 170mg |
|---|---|---|---|---|
| Pott: 280mg | Calcium: 160mg | Phos: 140mg | Fiber: 7g | Sugar: 11g |

## 4.16 CHIA BERRY PANCAKES

| PREPARATION TIME | COOKING TIME | SERVING |
|---|---|---|
| 10 mins | 15 mins | 2 |

### INGREDIENTS
1 cup whole wheat flour
¼ cup chia seeds
1 tsp baking powder
½ cup mixed berries (strawberries, blueberries, raspberries)
1 cup unsweetened almond milk
1 egg
1 tsp honey (optional)

### DIRECTIONS
1. Dry mixture preparation: Combine whole wheat flour, chia seeds, and yeast in a bowl.
2. Wet mixture preparation: In a separate bowl, whisk together almond milk and an egg until smooth.
3. Mixing the batters: Add the wet mixture to the dry mixture, stirring until well combined. Gently fold in mixed berries.
4. Cooking: Lightly oil a non-stick skillet and heat it over medium heat. Pour about 1/4 cup of batter for each pancake, cook until bubbles form on the surface, then flip and continue cooking until both sides are golden brown.

### Nutritional facts /value (per serving)
| Cal: 350 | Carbs: 50g | Protein: 10g | Total Fats: 9g | Sodium: 160mg |
|---|---|---|---|---|
| Pott: 340mg | Calcium: 220mg | Phos: 200mg | Fiber: 11g | Sugar: 11g |

## 4.17 SPINACH AND MUSHROOM PANCAKES

| PREPARATION TIME | COOKING TIME | SERVING |
|---|---|---|
| 10 mins | 15 mins | 2 |

### INGREDIENTS
1 cup whole wheat flour
¼ cup fresh spinach, chopped
¼ cup mushrooms, sliced
½ tsp olive oil
½ tsp garlic powder
½ tsp onion powder
Salt to taste
Pepper to taste
1 cup water or vegetable broth
1 egg

### DIRECTIONS
1. 
2. Begin by heating olive oil in a pan over medium heat. Add mushrooms and chopped spinach, and sauté them for approximately 4 minutes. Add a pinch of salt, onion powder, pepper, and garlic powder for added flavor.
3. In a mixing bowl, combine the cooked mushrooms, spinach, egg, and vegetable broth.

4. Grease a non-stick skillet with a small amount of oil and place it over medium heat.

5. To create the pancakes, ladle approximately 1/4 cup portions of the batter onto the heated griddle.

6. Cook until you observe bubbles forming on the surface, then flip and continue cooking until both sides achieve a delightful golden-brown color

### Nutritional facts /value (per serving)

| Cal: 210 | Carbs: 38g | Protein: 10g | Total Fats: 3g | Sodium: 380mg |
|---|---|---|---|---|
| Pott: 270mg | Calcium: 160mg | Phos: 180mg | Fiber: 6g | Sugar: 1g |

## 4.18 PUMPKIN SPICE WAFFLES

| PREPARATION TIME | COOKING TIME | SERVING |
|---|---|---|
| 15 mins | 20 mins | 2 |

### INGREDIENTS

1 cup whole wheat flour
¼ cup pumpkin puree, canned
1 tsp pumpkin pie spice
½ tsp baking powder
½ tsp vanilla extract
½ cup unsweetened almond milk
1 egg
1 tsp honey (optional)

### DIRECTIONS

1. In a mixing bowl, combine whole wheat flour, pumpkin pie seasoning, baking powder, and pumpkin pie spice.

2. In a separate bowl, whisk together almond milk, vanilla extract, and an egg until they are thoroughly blended.

3. Pour the wet ingredients into the dry mixture and stir until well combined. Gently fold in the mixed berries for a burst of flavor.

4. Grease a non-stick pan with a small amount of oil and place it over medium heat.

5. To create your pancakes, pour approximately 1/4 cup portions of the batter onto the heated griddle.

6. Cook until you observe bubbles forming on the surface, then carefully flip and continue cooking until both sides achieve a delightful golden-brown hue

### Nutritional facts /value (per serving)

| Cal: 270 | Carbs: 51g | Protein: 10g | Total Fats: 4g | Sodium: 190mg |
|---|---|---|---|---|
| Pott: 260mg | Calcium: 160mg | Phos: 160mg | Fiber: 8g | Sugar: 6g |

## 4.19 AVOCADO AND SPINACH BREAKFAST SALAD

| PREPARATION TIME | COOKING TIME | SERVING |
|---|---|---|
| 10 mins | 0 mins | 1 |

| INGREDIENTS | DIRECTIONS |
|---|---|
| 4 cups fresh spinach leaves<br>1 ripe avocado, sliced<br>2 boiled eggs, sliced<br>¼ cup cherry tomatoes, halved<br>¼ cup cucumber, chopped<br>2 tbsp pumpkin seeds<br>2 tbsp olive oil<br>1 tbsp lemon juice | 1. In a large mixing bowl, combine fresh spinach leaves, sliced avocado, boiled egg slices, cherry tomatoes, and chopped cucumber.<br>2. Create the dressing by mixing together olive oil, lemon juice, a pinch of salt, ground pepper, and a sprinkling of pumpkin seeds.<br>3. Drizzle the dressing over the salad ingredients and toss everything together until well coated. |

### Nutritional facts /value (per serving)

| Cal: 350 | Carbs: 16g | Protein: 10g | Total Fats: 28g | Sodium: 230mg |
|---|---|---|---|---|
| Pott: 900mg | Calcium: 160mg | Phos: 140mg | Fiber: 9g | Sugar: 3g |

## 4.20 GREEK BREAKFAST SALAD

| PREPARATION TIME | COOKING TIME | SERVING |
|---|---|---|
| 15 mins | 0 mins | 2 |

| INGREDIENTS | DIRECTIONS |
|---|---|
| 2 cups mixed greens (e.g., spinach, arugula, romaine)<br>½ cup cherry tomatoes, halved<br>½ cucumber, diced<br>¼ cup Kalamata olives, pitted and sliced<br>¼ cup crumbled feta cheese<br>2 boiled eggs, sliced<br>2 tbsp extra-virgin olive oil<br>1 tbsp red wine vinegar<br>½ tsp dried oregano | 1. Take a bowl and add mixed greens, Cherry tomatoes, diced cucumber, olives, feta cheese and boiled egg.<br>2. For dressing mix olive oil, red wine vinegar, dried oregano, salt and pepper<br>3. Pour dressing over salad and mix well.<br>4. Salad is ready to serve |

### Nutritional facts /value (per serving)

| Cal:340 | Carbs: 12g | Protein: 11g | Total Fats: 28g | Sodium: 720mg |
|---|---|---|---|---|
| Pott: 410mg | Calcium: 150mg | Phos: 140mg | Fiber: 4g | Sugar: 5g |

# 5. LUNCH RECIPES

## 5.1 SPINACH AND BEET SALAD

| PREPARATION TIME | COOKING TIME | SERVING |
|---|---|---|
| 15 mins | 5 mins | 4 |

| INGREDIENTS | DIRECTIONS |
|---|---|
| 6 cups baby spinach leaves<br>2 medium beets, roasted and sliced<br>¼ cup goat cheese, crumbled<br>¼ cup walnuts, chopped<br>¼ cup red onion, sliced<br>3 tbsp olive oil<br>2 tbsp fresh lemon juice<br>1 tsp honey (optional) | 1. For salad, mix baby spinach, sliced roasted beets, crumbled goat cheese, chopped walnuts, and sliced red onion.<br>2. For dressing, mix lemon juice, honey, salt, pepper and olive oil pour the dressing on the salad and gently toss to mix.<br>3. Salad is ready to serve. |

**Nutritional facts /value (per serving)**

| Cal: 200 | Carbs: 13g | Protein: 5g | Total Fats: 15g | Sodium: 160mg |
|---|---|---|---|---|
| Pott: 450mg | Calcium: 50mg | Phos: 130mg | Fiber: 4g | Sugar: 6g |

## 5.2 QUINOA AND CHICKPEA SALAD WITH TAHINI

| PREPARATION TIME | COOKING TIME | SERVING |
|---|---|---|
| 15 mins | 5 mins | 4 |

| INGREDIENTS | DIRECTIONS |
|---|---|
| 1 cup quinoa, cooked<br>1 can (15 oz) chickpeas, drained and rinsed<br>1 cup cherry tomatoes, halved<br>½ cucumber, diced<br>¼ cup fresh parsley, chopped<br>¼ cup feta cheese (optional), crumbled<br>3 tbsp tahini<br>2 tbsp fresh lemon juice<br>1 clove garlic, minced<br>2 tbsp water | 1. For salad take a large bowl and mix cooked quinoa, chickpeas, cherry tomato diced cucumber, chopped fresh parsley and crumbled feta cheese.<br>2. For dressing mix tahini, lemon juice, minced garlic, water, salt and pepper<br>3. Pour the dressing on the salad and gently toss to mix.<br>4. Salad is ready to serve. |

**Nutritional facts /value (per serving)**

| Cal: 300 | Carbs: 40g | Protein: 10g | Total Fats: 12g | Sodium: 290mg |
|---|---|---|---|---|
| Pott: 450mg | Calcium: 90mg | Phos: 160mg | Fiber: 8g | Sugar: 4g |

## 5.3 KALE SALAD WITH AVOCADO AND LIME DRESSING

| PREPARATION TIME | COOKING TIME | SERVING |
|---|---|---|
| 15 mins | 5 mins | 4 |

| INGREDIENTS | DIRECTIONS |
|---|---|
| 6 cups kale leaves, chopped<br>1 cup red cabbage, shredded<br>1 cup carrots, shredded<br>½ cup cherry tomatoes, halved<br>¼ cup pumpkin seeds<br>¼ cup cranberries, dried<br>1 ripe avocado, ripe<br>Juice of 2 limes<br>2 tbsp olive oil<br>1 clove garlic, minced | 1. For salad take a large bowl and mix chopped kale leaves, carrots, cabbage cherry tomatoes, pumpkin seeds, dried cranberries.<br>2. For dressing take a blender and blend avocado lime juice, minced garlic, salt and pepper<br>3. Pour the dressing on the salad and gently toss to mix.<br>4. Salad is ready to serve. |

**Nutritional facts /value (per serving)**

| Cal: 220 | Carbs: 23g | Protein: 6g | Total Fats: 14g | Sodium: 80 mg |
|---|---|---|---|---|
| Pott: 680mg | Calcium: 100mg | Phos: 130mg | Fiber: 6g | Sugar: 7g |

## 5.4 ROASTED VEGETABLE SALAD WITH BALSAMIC VINEGAR

| PREPARATION TIME | COOKING TIME | SERVING |
|---|---|---|
| 20 mins | 5 mins | 4 |

| INGREDIENTS | DIRECTIONS |
|---|---|
| 4 cups mixed vegetables (zucchini, bell peppers, eggplant, etc.), roasted<br>2 cups mixed greens<br>¼ cup goat cheese, crumbled<br>¼ cup fresh basil, chopped<br>¼ cup roasted nuts (almonds, walnuts), chopped<br>3 tbsp balsamic vinegar<br>2 tbsp olive oil<br>1 tsp Dijon mustard<br>1 tsp honey (optional) | 1. In a large bowl, combine mixed roasted vegetables, mixed greens, crumbled goat cheese, chopped fresh basil, and chopped roasted nuts.<br>2. For dressing mix vinegar, olive oil, Dijon mustard, honey, salt and pepper.<br>3. Pour dressing over the salad and serve. |

**Nutritional facts /value (per serving)**

| Cal: 250 | Carbs: 16g | Protein: 6g | Total Fats: 18g | Sodium: 260mg |
|---|---|---|---|---|
| Pott: 480mg | Calcium: 90mg | Phos: 120mg | Fiber: 6g | Sugar: 7g |

## 5.5    CITRUS AVOCADO SALAD WITH ORANGE

| PREPARATION TIME | COOKING TIME | SERVING |
|---|---|---|
| 15 mins | 5 mins | 4 |

### INGREDIENTS

6 cups mixed greens
2 oranges, peeled and segmented
1 avocado, sliced
¼ cup red onion, thinly sliced
¼ cup feta cheese (optional), crumbled
2 tbsp pine nuts, roasted
Juice of 2 oranges
2 tbsp olive oil
1 tsp honey (optional)

### DIRECTIONS

1. In a large bowl combine mixed greens orange segments, sliced avocado, thinly sliced red onion, crumbled feta cheese (if using), and toasted pine nuts.
2. For dressing mix vinegar, olive oil, juice of 2 oranges, honey, salt and pepper.
3. Pour dressing over the salad and serve

**Nutritional facts /value (per serving)**

| Cal: 280 | Carbs: 24g | Protein: 5g | Total Fats: 20g | Sodium: 190mg |
|---|---|---|---|---|
| Pott: 550mg | Calcium: 120mg | Phos: 70mg | Fiber: 6g | Sugar: 15g |

## 5.6    GRILLED CHICKEN AND STRAWBERRY SALAD

| PREPARATION TIME | COOKING TIME | SERVING |
|---|---|---|
| 20 mins | 5 mins | 4 |

### INGREDIENTS

2 boneless, skinless chicken breasts, grilled and sliced
6 cups mixed greens
1 cup strawberries, sliced
¼ cup goat cheese, crumbled
¼ cup fresh mint leaves, chopped
¼ cup pecans, chopped
3 tbsp balsamic glaze
2 tbsp olive oil
1 tsp honey (optional)

### DIRECTIONS

1. In a large bowl combine grilled chicken, mixed greens, strawberries, cheese, mint leaves and chopped pecans.
2. For dressing mix vinegar, olive oil, honey, salt and pepper.
3. Pour dressing over the salad and serve.

**Nutritional facts /value (per serving)**

| Cal: 310 | Carbs: 17g | Protein: 26g | Total Fats: 16g | Sodium: 260mg |
|---|---|---|---|---|
| Pott: 570mg | Calcium: 120mg | Phos: 250mg | Fiber: 4g | Sugar: 9g |

## 5.7    GRILLED CHICKEN AND AVOCADO WRAP

| PREPARATION TIME | COOKING TIME | SERVING |
|---|---|---|
| 15 mins | 0 mins | 2 |

| INGREDIENTS | DIRECTIONS |
|---|---|
| 2 whole wheat or spinach wraps<br>2 grilled chicken breasts, sliced<br>1 avocado, sliced<br>1 cup mixed greens<br>¼ cup red onion, sliced<br>¼ cup Greek yogurt<br>1 tbsp fresh lime juice | 1. Mix lime juice fresh yogurt, salt and pepper to make a sauce<br>2. Spread a tbsp of sauce on each wrap.<br>3. Divide the sliced grilled chicken, avocado slices, mixed greens, and sliced red onion evenly between the wraps.<br>4. Roll up the wraps and serve. |

**Nutritional facts /value (per serving)**

| Cal: 350 | Carbs: 24g | Protein: 25g | Total Fats: 18g | Sodium: 280mg |
|---|---|---|---|---|
| Pott: 720mg | Calcium: 70mg | Phos: 280mg | Fiber: 9g | Sugar: 3g |

## 5.8    MEDITERRANEAN HUMMUS WRAP

| PREPARATION TIME | COOKING TIME | SERVING |
|---|---|---|
| 10 mins | 0 mins | 2 |

| INGREDIENTS | DIRECTIONS |
|---|---|
| 2 whole wheat wraps ½ cup hummus<br>1 cup cucumber, chopped<br>1 cup tomatoes, diced<br>½ cup Kalamata olives, olives<br>¼ cup feta cheese (optional), crumbled<br>Fresh parsley, for garnish<br>Olive oil and lemon juice for drizzling<br>Salt to taste<br>Black pepper to taste | 1. Put hummus on each wrap and spread it evenly<br>2. Put diced cucumbers, tomatoes, olives, cheese on each wrap.<br>3. Put some drops of olive oil and season it with salt and pepper.<br>4. Roll up the wraps and serve. |

**Nutritional facts /value (per serving)**

| Cal: 350 | Carbs: 45g | Protein: 11g | Total Fats: 16g | Sodium: 650mg |
|---|---|---|---|---|
| Pott: 380mg | Calcium: 120mg | Phos: 150mg | Fiber: 8g | Sugar: 4g |

## 5.9    TURKEY AND CRANBERRY SANDWICH

| PREPARATION TIME | COOKING TIME | SERVING |
|---|---|---|
| 10 mins | 0 mins | 2 |

| INGREDIENTS | DIRECTIONS |
|---|---|
| 4 slices whole grain bread<br>8 oz turkey breast slices<br>¼ cup cranberry sauce<br>2 cups mixed greens<br>¼ cup red onion, sliced<br>2 tbsp Greek yogurt<br>1 tsp Dijon mustard<br>Salt to taste<br>Black pepper to taste | 1. To make a sauce mix yogurt, Dijon mustard, salt, and pepper.<br>2. Layer out the bread slices and put yogurt sauce on each slice.<br>3. Divide turkey breast slices, cranberry sauce, mixed greens, and red onion evenly between 2 of the bread slices.<br>4. Put other slice of bread on top<br>5. Turkey sandwich is ready to serve. |

### Nutritional facts /value (per serving)

| Cal: 350 | Carbs: 75g | Protein: 25g | Total Fats: 7g | Sodium: 600mg |
|---|---|---|---|---|
| Pott: 300mg | Calcium: 90mg | Phos: 230mg | Fiber: 7g | Sugar: 16g |

## 5.10    ROASTED VEGETABLE AND HUMMUS WRAP

| PREPARATION TIME | COOKING TIME | SERVING |
|---|---|---|
| 20 mins | 0 mins | 2 |

| INGREDIENTS | DIRECTIONS |
|---|---|
| 2 whole wheat wraps<br>1 cup vegetables (zucchini, bell peppers, eggplant, etc.), roasted<br>½ cup hummus<br>¼ cup goat cheese (optional), crumbled<br>Fresh basil leaves, for garnish<br>Olive oil and balsamic vinegar for drizzling | 1. Put generous amount of hummus on wraps and spread it.<br>2. Put roasted vegetables and crumbled cheese on each wrap.<br>3. Drizzle some vinegar and olive oil and season with salt and pepper. |

### Nutritional facts /value (per serving)

| Cal: 330 | Carbs: 37g | Protein: 10g | Total Fats: 16g | Sodium: 400mg |
|---|---|---|---|---|
| Pott: 470mg | Calcium: 60mg | Phos: 190mg | Fiber: 6g | Sugar: 3g |

## 5.11    LETTUCE AND EGG WRAP

| PREPARATION TIME | COOKING TIME | SERVING |
|---|---|---|
| 15 mins | 0 mins | 2 |

| INGREDIENTS | DIRECTIONS |
|---|---|
| 4 large lettuce leaves (e.g., iceberg or Romaine)<br>4 hard-boiled eggs, chopped<br>¼ cup Greek yogurt<br>2 tbsp Dijon mustard<br>¼ cup celery, diced<br>¼ cup red onion, diced<br><br>Paprika for garnish (optional) | 1. Begin by taking a bowl and combining chopped hard-boiled eggs, yogurt, Dijon mustard, diced celery, and diced onion. Mix these ingredients thoroughly, and season with a pinch of salt and a dash of pepper.<br>2. Lay out the fresh lettuce leaves on a clean surface.<br>3. Place a portion of the egg mixture onto each lettuce leaf and lightly sprinkle with paprika for added flavor.<br>4. Fold the lettuce leaves around the mixture to create delightful wraps |

### Nutritional facts /value (per serving)

| Cal: 270 | Carbs: 7g | Protein: 17g | Total Fats: 18g | Sodium: 370mg |
|---|---|---|---|---|
| Pott: 280mg | Calcium: 100mg | Phos: 240mg | Fiber: 1g | Sugar: 4g |

## 5.12    SMOKED SALMON AND CUCUMBER SANDWICH

| PREPARATION TIME | COOKING TIME | SERVING |
|---|---|---|
| 15 mins | 0 mins | 2 |

| INGREDIENTS | DIRECTIONS |
|---|---|
| 4 slices whole grain bread<br>4 oz salmon, smoked<br>½ cucumber, thinly sliced<br>¼ cup whipped cream cheese<br>1 tsp fresh dill, chopped<br>1 tsp lemon zest<br>Salt to taste<br>Black pepper to taste | 1. To make a sauce mix whipped cream cheese, chopped fresh dill, lemon zest, salt, and pepper<br>2. Layer out the bread slices and put whipped cream mixture on each slice.<br>3. Put smoked salmon and sliced cucumber between 2 of the bread slices<br>4. To create a sandwich, place the other slice of bread on top. |

### Nutritional facts /value (per serving)

| Cal: 280 | Carbs: 35g | Protein: 16g | Total Fats: 10g | Sodium: 660mg |
|---|---|---|---|---|
| Pott: 340mg | Calcium: 100mg | Phos: 200mg | Fiber: 5g | Sugar: 7g |

## *5.13   QUINOA AND ROASTED VEGETABLE BOWL*

| PREPARATION TIME | COOKING TIME | SERVING |
|---|---|---|
| 20 mins | 20 mins | 2 |

### INGREDIENTS

1 cup cooked quinoa
2 cups mixed roasted vegetables (such as zucchini, bell peppers, eggplant, etc.)
¼ cup crumbled feta cheese (optional)
¼ cup chopped fresh basil
2 tbsp balsamic glaze
Salt, to taste
Pepper, to taste

### DIRECTIONS

1. Begin by selecting a bowl and placing the cooked quinoa in it.
2. Add a medley of roasted vegetables and crumbled cheese to the bowl with the quinoa.
3. Enhance the flavors by drizzling balsamic vinegar, adding fresh basil leaves, and seasoning with a pinch of salt and a dash of pepper.

### Nutritional facts /value (per serving)

| Cal: 350 | Carbs: 52g | Protein: 9g | Total Fats: 10g | Sodium: 290mg |
|---|---|---|---|---|
| Pott: 560mg | Calcium: 90mg | Phos: 230mg | Fiber: 7g | Sugar: 5g |

## *5.14   SPINACH AND LENTIL PILAF*

| PREPARATION TIME | COOKING TIME | SERVING |
|---|---|---|
| 25 mins | 25 mins | 2 |

### INGREDIENTS

1 cup brown rice, cooked
½ cup green or brown lentils, cooked
2 cups fresh spinach leaves
¼ cup red onion, diced
¼ cup fresh parsley, chopped
2 tbsp lemon juice
2 tbsp olive oil
Salt to taste
Pepper to taste

### DIRECTIONS

1. Mix cooked rice and cooked lentils in a bowl.
2. Add fresh spinach leave, parsley and red onion.
3. Add lemon juice, olive oil, and toss to combine.

### Nutritional facts /value (per serving)

| Cal: 300 | Carbs: 45g | Protein: 12g | Total Fats: 10g | Sodium: 30mg |
|---|---|---|---|---|
| Pott: 570mg | Calcium: 60mg | Phos: 230mg | Fiber: 10g | Sugar: 2g |

## *5.15* *MEDITERRANEAN QUINOA BOWL*

| PREPARATION TIME | COOKING TIME | SERVING |
|---|---|---|
| 20 mins | 30 mins | 2 |

| INGREDIENTS | DIRECTIONS |
|---|---|
| 1 cup quinoa, cooked<br>1 cup chickpeas, cooked or canned<br>1 cup cucumber, diced<br>½ cup cherry tomatoes, halved<br>¼ cup Kalamata sliced olives<br>¼ cup feta cheese (optional), crumbled<br>Fresh parsley leaves, for garnish<br>Olive oil and lemon juice for drizzling | 1. Take a bowl, add cooked quinoa and cooked chickpeas<br>2. Add diced cucumber, cherry tomatoes, olives, cheese in it.<br>3. Add lemon juice and oil over the mixture, then season with salt and pepper.<br>4. Garnish with fresh parsley leaves. |

**Nutritional facts /value (per serving)**

| Cal: 350 | Carbs: 51.1g | Protein: 12.3g | Total Fats: 12g | Sodium: 540mg |
|---|---|---|---|---|
| Pott: 670mg | Calcium: 100mg | Phos: 240mg | Fiber: 9g | Sugar: 4g |

## *5.16* *BARLEY AND CHICKPEA BOWL*

| PREPARATION TIME | COOKING TIME | SERVING |
|---|---|---|
| 25 mins | 25 mins | 2 |

| INGREDIENTS | DIRECTIONS |
|---|---|
| 1 cup barley, cooked<br>1 cup chickpeas, cooked<br>½ cup cucumber, diced<br>½ cup red bell pepper, diced<br>¼ cup fresh mint leaves, chopped<br>¼ cup dried apricots, chopped<br>¼ cup almonds, chopped<br>2 tbsp tahini<br>Juice of 1 lemon<br>1 clove garlic, minced<br>2 tbsp water | 1. Mixed cooked barley and cooked chickpeas.<br>2. Add diced cucumber, bell pepper, dried apricot, fresh mint leaves and chopped almonds.<br>3. Mix tahini, lemon juice, minced garlic, water, salt and pepper to make dressing<br>4. Put dressing over the bowl and mix. |

**Nutritional facts /value (per serving)**

| Cal: 370 | Carbs: 59g | Protein: 11g | Total Fats: 12g | Sodium: 270mg |
|---|---|---|---|---|
| Pott: 470mg | Calcium: 80mg | Phos: 210mg | Fiber: 10g | Sugar: 11g |

## 5.17   QUINOA AND LEMON HERB PILAF

| PREPARATION TIME | COOKING TIME | SERVING |
|---|---|---|
| 20 mins | 20 mins | 2 |

| INGREDIENTS | DIRECTIONS |
|---|---|
| 1 cup quinoa, cooked<br>¼ cup fresh parsley, chopped<br>¼ cup fresh cilantro, chopped<br>¼ cup fresh mint leaves, chopped<br>2 tbsp lemon juice<br>2 tbsp olive oil<br>1 clove garlic, minced | 1. Mix cooked quinoa with freshly chopped parsley, cilantro, and mint leaves in a bowl.<br>2. Create a zesty dressing in a separate small bowl by whisking together lemon juice, olive oil, minced garlic, salt, and pepper.<br>3. Drizzle the dressing over the quinoa mixture and toss everything together until well combined. |

**Nutritional facts /value (per serving)**

| Cal: 240 | Carbs: 29g | Protein: 5g | Total Fats: 12g | Sodium: 15mg |
|---|---|---|---|---|
| Pott: 200mg | Calcium: 30mg | Phos: 90mg | Fiber: 4g | Sugar: 1g |

## 5.18   MUSHROOM PILAF

| PREPARATION TIME | COOKING TIME | SERVING |
|---|---|---|
| 10 mins | 30 mins | 1 |

| INGREDIENTS | DIRECTIONS |
|---|---|
| 1 cup wild rice, cooked<br>1 cup mushrooms, sliced<br>¼ cup onion, diced<br>2 cloves garlic, minced<br>2 tbsp fresh thyme, chopped<br>2 tbsp olive oil | 1. Take a pan, heat olive oil over medium heat. Add diced onion and minced garlic. Cook for a few minutes.<br>2. Add mushrooms and fresh thyme in the pan. Cook for 5 more minutes.<br>3. Mix cooked rice and mushroom mixture. |

**Nutritional facts /value (per serving)**

| Cal: 250 | Carbs: 35g | Protein: 6g | Total Fats: 10g | Sodium:10mg |
|---|---|---|---|---|
| Pott: 290mg | Calcium: 20mg | Phos: 150mg | Fiber: 3g | Sugar: 2g |

## 5.19    VEGETABLE AND CHICKEN SOUP

| PREPARATION TIME | COOKING TIME | SERVING |
|---|---|---|
| 20 mins | 30 mins | 4 |

| INGREDIENTS | DIRECTIONS |
|---|---|
| 1 lb. b1less, skinless chicken breast, cubed<br>4 cups low-sodium chicken broth<br>2 carrots, sliced<br>2 celery stalks, sliced<br>1 onion, chopped<br>2 cloves garlic, minced<br>1 cup green beans, chopped<br>1 cup spinach leaves<br>1 tsp thyme, dried<br><br>Fresh parsley, for garnish | 1. Take a big pot, sauté the onion and garlic for 5 minutes until light golden<br>2. Add chicken, carrots, celery, and green beans. Cook for a few minutes until the chicken changes its color<br>3. Add chicken broth and dried thyme. cook for about 20 minutes.<br>4. Add spinach leaves and cook for 5 more minutes.<br>5. Season with salt and pepper and garnish with fresh parsley. |

### Nutritional facts /value (per serving)

| Cal: 180 | Carbs: 12g | Protein: 25g | Total Fats: 3g | Sodium: 330mg |
|---|---|---|---|---|
| Pott: 690mg | Calcium: 60mg | Phos: 230mg | Fiber: 3g | Sugar: 4g |

## 5.20    VEGETABLE AND LENTIL STEW

| PREPARATION TIME | COOKING TIME | SERVING |
|---|---|---|
| 15 mins | 40 mins | 4 |

| INGREDIENTS | DIRECTIONS |
|---|---|
| 1 cup dried green or brown lentils, dried<br>4 cups vegetable broth<br>2 carrots, diced<br>2 celery stalks, diced<br>1 onion, chopped<br>2 cloves garlic, minced<br>1 cup tomatoes (canned or fresh), diced<br>1 tsp cumin, powder<br>1 tsp paprika<br><br>Fresh cilantro for garnishing | 1. In a pot, place the onions and garlic, and cook them for approximately 5 to 6 minutes until they turn a light golden color and release their aromatic fragrance.<br>2. Introduce the diced carrots and celery into the pot, and cook for a few minutes until they start to soften.<br>3. Combine vegetable broth, lentils, tomatoes, cumin, and paprika in the pot. Allow the mixture to simmer for about 30-35 minutes, or until the lentils have softened.<br>4. Season the dish with   and garnish it with fresh cilantro. |

### Nutritional facts /value (per serving)

| Cal: 220 | Carbs: 39g | Protein: 14g | Total Fats: 1g | Sodium: 490mg |
|---|---|---|---|---|
| Pott: 730mg | Calcium: 40mg | Phos: 230mg | Fiber: 16g | Sugar: 6g |

## 5.21 WHITE BEAN AND SPINACH SOUP

| PREPARATION TIME | COOKING TIME | SERVING |
|---|---|---|
| 15 mins | 30 mins | 4 |

### INGREDIENTS

1 can (15 oz) white beans
4 cups vegetable broth
1 onion, chopped
2 cloves garlic, minced
4 cups spinach leaves
1 tsp Italian seasoning, dried
Salt to taste
Pepper to taste
Grated Parmesan cheese (optional)

### DIRECTIONS

1. Put garlic and onion in a saucepan and cook for 5 to 6 minutes until it becomes light golden and aromatic,
2. Add white beans, spinach, vegetable broth and Italian seasoning and cook for 25 minutes.
3. Add salt and pepper and serve with grated parmesan cheese.

**Nutritional facts /value (per serving)**

| Cal: 160 | Carbs: 30g | Protein: 9g | Total Fats: 1g | Sodium: 580mg |
|---|---|---|---|---|
| Pott: 720mg | Calcium: 80mg | Phos: 120mg | Fiber: 8g | Sugar: 4g |

## 5.22 RICE AND TURKEY SOUP

| PREPARATION TIME | COOKING TIME | SERVING |
|---|---|---|
| 20 mins | 25 mins | 4 |

### INGREDIENTS

1 lb. ground turkey
4 cups chicken broth
1 cup white or brown rice, cooked
2 carrots, sliced
2 celery stalks, sliced
1 onion, chopped
2 cloves garlic, minced
1 tsp dried thyme
Salt to taste
Black pepper to taste
Fresh dill, for garnish

### DIRECTIONS

1. In a large pot, brown the ground turkey. Then, add the chopped onion and garlic, cooking for a few minutes until they become fragrant.
2. Incorporate the chicken broth, carrots, celery, and dried thyme into the pot. Cook for approximately 20 minutes or until the vegetables have softened.
3. Add the cooked rice to the mixture and continue cooking for an additional 5 minutes.
4. Season the dish with salt and pepper according to your taste, and garnish it with freshly chopped dill.

**Nutritional facts /value (per serving)**

| Cal: 230 | Carbs: 24.1g | Protein: 21g | Total Fats: 6g | Sodium: 330mg |
|---|---|---|---|---|
| Pott: 600mg | Calcium: 60mg | Phos: 180mg | Fiber: 3g | Sugar: 4g |

## 5.23   TOMATO AND LENTIL SOUP

| PREPARATION TIME | COOKING TIME | SERVING |
|---|---|---|
| 15 mins | 30 mins | 4 |

| INGREDIENTS | DIRECTIONS |
|---|---|
| 1 cup red lentils, dried<br>4 cups low-sodium vegetable broth<br>1 onion, chopped<br>2 cloves garlic, minced<br>1 can (15 oz) tomatoes, diced<br>1 tsp g cumin, ground<br>1 tsp paprika<br><br>Fresh cilantro, for garnish | 1. Place chopped onion and garlic into a pot and cook for approximately 5 to 6 minutes until they release their aromatic fragrance.<br><br>2. Introduce lentils, vegetable broth, tomatoes, cumin, and paprika into the pot and allow them to simmer for 20 to 25 minutes.<br><br>3. Season the dish with salt and black pepper to your liking.<br><br>4. Just before serving, garnish the dish with a sprinkle of fresh cilantro. |

### Nutritional facts /value (per serving)

| Cal: 230 | Carbs: 38g | Protein: 15g | Total Fats: 1g | Sodium: 680mg |
|---|---|---|---|---|
| Pott: 580mg | Calcium: 60mg | Phos: 230mg | Fiber: 11g | Sugar: 4g |

## 5.24   BUTTERNUT SQUASH AND APPLE SOUP

| PREPARATION TIME | COOKING TIME | SERVING |
|---|---|---|
| 20 mins | 35 mins | 4 |

| INGREDIENTS | DIRECTIONS |
|---|---|
| 1 butternut squash, peeled, seeded, and diced<br>2 apples, peeled, cored, and diced<br>1 onion, chopped<br>4 cups low-sodium vegetable broth<br>1 tsp ground cinnamon<br>½ tsp ground nutmeg<br><br>Greek yogurt (optional, for garnish) | 1. In a spacious pot, place the chopped onion and sauté until it undergoes a change in color.<br><br>2. Introduce butternut squash, apples, vegetable broth, ground cinnamon, and ground nutmeg into the pot. Simmer for approximately 25-30 minutes, or until the squash and apples have reached a tender state.<br><br>3. Utilize a blender to puree the soup until it achieves a smooth consistency. Season the soup with salt and pepper to your preference. Optionally, serve it with a dollop of Greek yogurt. |

### Nutritional facts /value (per serving)

| Cal: 170 | Carbs: 43g | Protein: 2g | Total Fats: 0.5g | Sodium: 320mg |
|---|---|---|---|---|
| Pott: 800mg | Calcium: 80mg | Phos: 70mg | Fiber: 8g | Sugar: 18g |

# 6. DINNER RECIPES

## 6.1    VEGETABLE AND QUINOA CASSEROLE

| PREPARATION TIME | COOKING TIME | SERVING |
|---|---|---|
| 30 mins | 45 mins | 6 |

| INGREDIENTS | DIRECTIONS |
|---|---|
| 1 cup uncooked quinoa<br>2 cups water<br>2 cups mixed chopped vegetables (e.g., broccoli, cauliflower, carrots)<br>1 cup low-fat cottage cheese<br>1/2 cup grated Parmesan cheese<br>1/4 cup chopped fresh basil<br>2 cloves minced garlic<br><br>1 cup optional shredded mozzarella cheese | 1. Preheat the oven to 375°F (190°C).<br>2. Boil quinoa for 15 minutes, then remove from heat.<br>3. In a large bowl, combine cooked quinoa, mixed vegetables, low-fat cottage cheese, grated Parmesan, fresh basil, minced garlic, salt, and pepper.<br>4. Transfer the mixture to a greased casserole dish. Optionally, top with shredded mozzarella.<br>5. Cover with foil and bake for 30 minutes. Remove the foil and bake for an additional 15 minutes until the casserole is golden and bubbling. |

### Nutritional facts /value (per serving)

| Cal: 220 | Carbs: 29g | Protein: 14g | Total Fats: 6g | Sodium: 330mg |
|---|---|---|---|---|
| Pott: 330mg | Calcium: 190mg | Phos: 180mg | Fiber: 4g | Sugar: 2g |

## 6.2    SWEET POTATO AND LENTIL PIE

| PREPARATION TIME | COOKING TIME | SERVING |
|---|---|---|
| 40 mins | 45 mins | 6 |

| INGREDIENTS | DIRECTIONS |
|---|---|
| 2 cups green or brown lentils, cooked<br>2 cups sweet potatoes, mashed<br>1 onion, chopped<br>2 cloves garlic, minced<br>2 carrots, diced<br>1 cup peas, frozen<br>1 cup vegetable broth<br>2 tbsp olive oil<br>1 tsp thyme, dried | 1. Preheat the oven to 375°F (190°C).<br>2. Take a skillet and sauté chopped onion, garlic, carrots, salt, pepper, and dried thyme in olive oil for 10 minutes.<br>3. Add lentils, frozen peas, and vegetable broth. Simmer for 5 minutes until the sauce thickens.<br>4. Transfer the mixture to a casserole dish and spread mashed sweet potato on top. Bake for 30-35 minutes. |

### Nutritional facts /value (per serving)

| Cal: 230 | Carbs: 43g | Protein: 10g | Total Fats: 4g | Sodium: 240mg |
|---|---|---|---|---|
| Pott: 570mg | Calcium: 50mg | Phos: 160mg | Fiber: 9g | Sugar: 6g |

## 6.3   EGGPLANT AND CHICKPEA CASSEROLE

| PREPARATION TIME | COOKING TIME | SERVING |
|---|---|---|
| 30 mins | 45 mins | 6 |

| INGREDIENTS | DIRECTIONS |
|---|---|
| 1 eggplant, cut into slices<br>30-ounce chickpeas<br>1 onion, chopped<br>2 cloves garlic, minced<br>1 can (14 oz) tomatoes, diced<br>1 tsp oregano, dried<br>½ tsp cumin, powder<br>Salt to taste<br> pepper to taste<br>2 cups tomato sauce (low-sodium)<br>1 cup low-fat mozzarella cheese (optional), shredded<br>Fresh basil leaves, for garnish | 1. Preheat the oven to 375°F (190°C).<br>2. Take a pan and add chopped onion, minced garlic, thinly sliced eggplant and cook until lightly browned. Remove from heat.<br>3. In a separate bowl, combine drained chickpeas, diced tomatoes, dried oregano, ground cumin, salt, and pepper.<br>4. Grease a casserole dish, layer half of the eggplant slices. add chickpea mixture on top, then layer the remaining eggplant slices.<br>5. Add tomato sauce over the casserole. Add mozzarella cheese if you like.<br>6. Cover with foil and bake for 40 minutes. Garnish with fresh basil leaves before serving. |

**Nutritional facts /value (per serving)**

| **Cal:** 220 | **Carbs:** 38g | **Protein:** 8.8g | **Total Fats:** 2.9g | **Sodium:** 330mg |
|---|---|---|---|---|
| **Pott:** 570mg | **Calcium:** 90mg | **Phos:** 170mg | **Fiber:** 10g | **Sugar:** 6g |

## 6.4   MUSHROOM AND TURKEY CASSEROLE

| PREPARATION TIME | COOKING TIME | SERVING |
|---|---|---|
| 30 mins | 30 mins | 6 |

| INGREDIENTS | DIRECTIONS |
|---|---|
| 1 lb. ground turkey<br>1 cup quinoa, uncooked<br>2 cups water<br>1 lb. mushrooms, sliced<br>1 onion, medium, cut into dices<br>2 garlic cloves, crushed<br>2 cups chicken broth, low sodium<br>1 cup plain Greek yogurt, low fat<br>¼ cup of parmesan cheese, shredded<br>1tsp dried thyme | 1. Begin by boiling thoroughly rinsed quinoa for 15 minutes.<br>2. In a skillet, cook ground turkey, onion, mushrooms, and garlic until the mushrooms achieve a browned appearance, and the onion turns translucent. Then, add dried thyme for added flavor.<br>3. Take a bowl and add the partially cooked quinoa, turkey-mushroom mix, yogurt, salt, pepper, and cheese. |

4. Transfer the mixture into a casserole dish and pour chicken broth over it.
5. Cover the dish with foil and bake for 20 minutes. After removing the foil, continue baking for an additional 10 minutes

### Nutritional facts /value (per serving)

| Cal: 290 | Carbs: 25g | Protein: 25g | Total Fats: 10g | Sodium: 240mg |
|---|---|---|---|---|
| Pott: 580mg | Calcium: 170mg | Phos: 310mg | Fiber: 3g | Sugar: 4g |

## 6.5    BROWN RICE AND SPINACH CASSEROLE

| PREPARATION TIME | COOKING TIME | SERVING |
|---|---|---|
| 30 mins | 45 mins | 6 |

### INGREDIENTS
2 cups brown rice, cooked
1 lb. fresh spinach leaves
1 onion, chopped
2 cloves garlic, minced
2 cups vegetable broth, low sodium
½ cup milk, low fat
¼ cup Parmesan cheese, grated
¼ cup low-fat cheddar cheese, shredded
¼ cup whole wheat breadcrumbs
2 tbsp olive oil
Fresh basil leaves, for garnish

### DIRECTIONS
1. Start by preheating the oven to 375°F (190°C).
2. In a spacious pan, heat olive oil and cook the onion, garlic, and spinach until the spinach wilts.
3. In a mixing bowl, combine the cooked rice, the spinach mixture, milk, cheese, salt, and pepper.
4. Take a separate bowl, add whole wheat breadcrumbs and more cheese.
5. Sprinkle the dry mixture evenly on the on the wet mixture.
6. Bake the dish for 25-30 minutes in a preheated oven.

### Nutritional facts /value (per serving)

| Cal: 220 | Carbs: 34g | Protein: 9g | Total Fats: 6g | Sodium: 330mg |
|---|---|---|---|---|
| Pott: 590mg | Calcium: 220mg | Phos: 200mg | Fiber: 3g | Sugar: 4g |

## 6.6   TUNA AND BEAN CASSEROLE

| PREPARATION TIME | COOKING TIME | SERVING |
|---|---|---|
| 30 mins | 30 mins | 6 |

| INGREDIENTS | DIRECTIONS |
|---|---|
| 2 tbsp of olive oil<br>2 cans (15 oz each) white beans<br>2 cans (5 oz each) tuna in water<br>1 onion, chopped<br>2 cloves garlic, minced<br>1 can (14 oz) tomatoes, diced<br>¼ cup low-fat plain Greek yogurt<br>¼ cup Parmesan cheese, grated<br>1 tsp basil, dried<br>A cup of whole wheat breadcrumbs | 1. Preheat the oven to 375°F (190°C).<br>2. Take a big pan and sauté onion and garlic for 2 minutes then add tomato, yogurt, drained tuna, drained beans, salt, pepper, and dried basil and stir to combine<br>3. Transfer his mixture into casserole dish. Bake for 25 to 30 minutes in the pre heated oven |

**Nutritional facts /value (per serving)**

| Cal: 280 | Carbs: 34g | Protein: 19g | Total Fats: 8g | Sodium: 360mg |
|---|---|---|---|---|
| Pott: 600mg | Calcium: 200mg | Phos: 370mg | Fiber: 10g | Sugar: 4g |

## 6.7   GRILLED SALMON WITH LEMON AND DILL

| PREPARATION TIME | COOKING TIME | SERVING |
|---|---|---|
| 10 mins | 10 mins | 4 |

| INGREDIENTS | DIRECTIONS |
|---|---|
| 4 salmon fillets (6 oz each)<br>2 lemons, thinly sliced<br>2 tbsp fresh dill, chopped<br>2 cloves garlic, minced<br>2 tbsp olive oil | 1. Preheat the grill to medium-high heat.<br>2. Take a small bowl, mix minced garlic, chopped fresh dill, olive oil, salt, and pepper. Marinate fish fillets with garlic mixture.<br>3. Top each fillet with lemon slices. Wrap the salmon in aluminum foil, sealing it properly.<br>4. Grill the salmon for about 10 minutes. |

**Nutritional facts /value (per serving)**

| Cal: 240 | Carbs: 4g | Protein: 34g | Total Fats: 9g | Sodium: 130mg |
|---|---|---|---|---|
| Pott: 430mg | Calcium: 30mg | Phos: 280mg | Fiber: 1g | Sugar: 1g |

## 6.8   MIXED GREENS AND TEMPEH

| PREPARATION TIME | COOKING TIME | SERVING |
|---|---|---|
| 15 mins | 15 mins | 4 |

### INGREDIENTS

1 block (14 oz) tempeh, cubed and pressed
2 cups mixed vegetables (broccoli, bell peppers, spinach etc.), chopped
2 cloves garlic, minced
1-inch piece of ginger, grated
¼ cup soy sauce or tamari
2 tbsp rice vinegar
1 tbsp sesame oil
1 tsp vegetable oil
Sesame seeds and sliced green onions, for garnish

### DIRECTIONS

1. Heat vegetable oil in a pan. Add cubed tempeh and cook until it's nicely browned on all sides. Remove the tempeh from the pan and set it aside.

2. In the same pan, add sesame oil, garlic, and ginger. Sauté for a minute until the aroma is fragrant.

3. Incorporate the mixed greens into the pan and stir-fry them for about 5-7 minutes.

4. In a separate bowl, combine low-sodium soy sauce and rice vinegar. Pour this sauce mixture into the pan with the sautéed vegetables.

5. Reintroduce the cooked tempeh to the pan and toss everything together to ensure it's well coated with the sauce.

### Nutritional facts /value (per serving)

| Cal: 200 | Carbs: 11g | Protein: 15g | Total Fats: 11g | Sodium: 680mg |
|---|---|---|---|---|
| Pott: 570mg | Calcium: 220mg | Phos: 190mg | Fiber: 4g | Sugar: 3g |

## 6.9   LEMON HERB CHICKEN BREAST

| PREPARATION TIME | COOKING TIME | SERVING |
|---|---|---|
| 10 mins | 30 mins | 4 |

### INGREDIENTS

4 b1less, skinless chicken breasts
2 lemons, juiced and zested
2 tbsp fresh rosemary, chopped
2 cloves garlic, minced
2 tbsp olive oil

Lemon wedges, for garnish

### DIRECTIONS

1. Set the oven temperature to 375°F (190°C).

2. In a small bowl, mix lemon juice, lemon zest, chopped rosemary, minced garlic, olive oil, salt, and pepper.

3. Marinate chicken with lemon mixture and bake for about 25-30

4. Use lemon wedges for garnishing.

### Nutritional facts /value (per serving)

| Cal: 240 | Carbs: 5.1g | Protein: 34g | Total Fats: 8.7g | Sodium: 130mg |
|---|---|---|---|---|
| Pott: 430mg | Calcium: 30mg | Phos: 280mg | Fiber: 1g | Sugar: 1g |

## 6.10   GARLIC SHRIMP WITH ZUCCHINI NOODLES

| PREPARATION TIME | COOKING TIME | SERVING |
|---|---|---|
| 15 mins | 10 mins | 4 |

### INGREDIENTS
1-pound large shrimp, peeled and deveined
4 medium zucchinis, spiralized into noodles
Juice and zest of 2 lemons
4 cloves of garlic, minced
2 tbsp olive oil
Salt and black pepper, to taste
Fresh parsley for garnish

### DIRECTIONS
1. In a pan, heat olive oil over medium heat. Add minced garlic and sauté for about a minute until it becomes fragrant.
2. Add the shrimp to the pan and cook for approximately 2-3 minutes on each side until they're cooked through. Once done, remove the shrimp from the pan and set them aside.
3. In the same pan, add the spiralized zucchini noodles and sauté them for about 2-3 minutes until they begin to soften.
4. Return the cooked shrimp to the skillet with the zucchini noodles.
5. Stir in lemon juice, lemon zest, salt, and pepper. Continue cooking for another minute until everything is thoroughly heated through.

### Nutritional facts /value (per serving)

| **Cal**: 190 | **Carbs**: 9.2g | **Protein**: 23g | **Total Fats**: 7.9g | **Sodium**: 170mg |
|---|---|---|---|---|
| **Pott**: 660mg | **Calcium**: 60mg | **Phos**: 200mg | **Fiber**: 2g | **Sugar**: 4g |

## 6.11   VEGGIE AND BAKED CHICKEN

| PREPARATION TIME | COOKING TIME | SERVING |
|---|---|---|
| 15 mins | 30 mins | 4 |

### INGREDIENTS
4 chicken breasts, b1less, skinless
2 cups mixed vegetables (zucchini, bell peppers, carrots, etc.), chopped
1 cup cherry tomatoes, halved
2 cloves garlic, minced
2 tbsp olive oil
1 tsp dried Italian seasoning
Salt
Pepper
Fresh basil leaves, for garnish

### DIRECTIONS
1. Set the oven temperature to 375°F (190°C).
2. Mix garlic, dried Italian seasoning, olive oil, salt, and pepper in a bowl.
3. Take 4 squares of aluminum foil. Place a chicken breast in the center of each foil square.
4. Put chopped mixed vegetables and cherry tomatoes evenly in the foil packets, placing them around the chicken.
5. Add garlic and herb mixture on each chicken breast and the vegetables.
6. Seal each foil packet properly.

7. Bake for 25-30 minutes until the chicken is cooked through and the vegetables are tender.

**Nutritional facts /value (per serving)**

| Cal: 240 | Carbs: 8g | Protein: 29g | Total Fats: 10g | Sodium: 90mg |
|---|---|---|---|---|
| Pott: 770mg | Calcium: 50mg | Phos: 260mg | Fiber: 3g | Sugar: 4g |

## 6.12   BELL PEPPERS STUFFED WITH LENTILS AND MUSHROOMS

| PREPARATION TIME | COOKING TIME | SERVING |
|---|---|---|
| 30 mins | 45 mins | 4 |

### INGREDIENTS

4 large bell peppers
1 cup brown lentils, uncooked
2 cups vegetable broth
1 cup mushrooms, chopped
1 onion, chopped
2 cloves garlic, minced
1 can (14 oz) tomatoes, diced
2 tbsp olive oil
1 tsp dried thyme, dried
Fresh parsley, for garnish

### DIRECTIONS

1. Begin by preheating your oven to 375°F (190°C).
2. Wash the lentils and place them in vegetable broth in a saucepan. Bring to a boil, then reduce the heat, cover, and cook the lentils for 20 to 25 minutes. Drain any excess liquid.
3. In a large skillet, heat oil over medium heat. Mix in chopped onion and mushrooms, cooking until the mushrooms soften and the onion turns translucent. Stir in garlic, salt, pepper, and thyme
4. Let it cook for another minute to be fragrant.
5. Incorporate the cooked lentils and diced tomatoes into the skillet. Cook for a few more minutes, allowing the flavors to meld.
6. Cut the tops off the bell peppers and stuff each bell pepper with the lentil and mushroom mixture.
7. Place the stuffed peppers in the preheated oven and bake for approximately 25-30 minutes, or until the peppers have become soft.

**Nutritional facts /value (per serving)**

| Cal: 270 | Carbs: 47g | Protein: 13g | Total Fats: 5g | Sodium: 520mg |
|---|---|---|---|---|
| Pott: 760mg | Calcium: 60mg | Phos: 240mg | Fiber: 14g | Sugar: 8g |

## 6.13 ACORN SQUASH STUFFED WITH MUSHROOM AND SPINACH

| PREPARATION TIME | COOKING TIME | SERVING |
|---|---|---|
| 20 mins | 45 mins | 4 |

### INGREDIENTS

2 acorn squashes, halved and seeds removed
2 cups spinach, chopped
2 cups mushrooms, chopped
1 onion, chopped
2 cloves garlic, minced
¼ cup Parmesan cheese (optional), grated
2 tbsp olive oil

Fresh thyme leaves, for garnish

### DIRECTIONS

1. Preheat the oven to 375°F (190°C).
2. Place the acorn squash halves on a baking sheet. Roast for about 30-35 minutes.
3. In a large pan heat olive oil. Add chopped onion and sauté until translucent.
4. Add garlic, mushrooms, and spinach. Cook until the mushrooms are soft and the spinach is wilted.
5. Fill each acorn half with the spinach and mushroom mixture.
6. Put the stuffed acorn squash in the oven and roast for an additional 10-15 minutes.

**Nutritional facts / value (per serving)**

| Cal: 160 | Carbs: 32g | Protein: 3g | Total Fats: 4g | Sodium: 15mg |
|---|---|---|---|---|
| Pott: 880mg | Calcium: 80mg | Phos: 100mg | Fiber: 5g | Sugar: 1g |

## 6.14 ROASTED VEGGIE AND CHICKPEA BOWL

| PREPARATION TIME | COOKING TIME | SERVING |
|---|---|---|
| 20 mins | 30 mins | 4 |

### INGREDIENTS

1 cup quinoa, uncooked
2 cups water
2 cups mixed vegetables (bell peppers, zucchini, cherry tomatoes, etc.), chopped
1 can (15 oz) chickpeas, drained and rinsed
2 tbsp olive oil
3 cloves garlic, crushed
1 tsp dried thyme
Juice of 1 lemon

### DIRECTIONS

1. Begin by washing the quinoa and boiling it for 15-20 minutes until it's fully cooked.
2. Preheat your oven to 425°F (220°C).
3. In a spacious bowl, combine chopped mixed vegetables and chickpeas with olive oil, pepper, minced garlic, salt, and dried thyme.
4. Spread the vegetable and chickpea mixture evenly on a baking sheet, then roast it for approximately 20-25 minutes.
5. To serve, layer the cooked quinoa with the roasted vegetable and chickpea mixture in a serving bowl.

**Nutritional facts / value (per serving)**

| Cal: 350 | Carbs: 59g | Protein: 12g | Total Fats: 8g | Sodium: 200mg |
|---|---|---|---|---|
| Pott: 640mg | Calcium: 60mg | Phos: 230mg | Fiber: 11g | Sugar: 5g |

## 6.15   ZUCCHINI AND TOMATO SAUTE

| PREPARATION TIME | COOKING TIME | SERVING |
|---|---|---|
| 10 mins | 10 mins | 2 |

| INGREDIENTS | DIRECTIONS |
|---|---|
| 2 medium zucchinis, sliced into rounds<br>1 cup cherry tomatoes, halved<br>2 cloves garlic, minced<br>1 tbsp olive oil | 1. In a large pan, heat olive oil over medium heat. Add minced garlic and cook for approximately 30 seconds until it becomes fragrant.<br>2. Introduce sliced zucchini rounds and halved cherry tomatoes to the pan. Sauté for about 5-7 minutes until the vegetables become tender and develop a slight caramelization.<br>3. Season the mixture with salt and pepper to your taste. |

**Nutritional facts /value (per serving)**

| Cal: 70 | Carbs: 7g | Protein: 2g | Total Fats: 5g | Sodium: 10mg |
|---|---|---|---|---|
| Pott: 350mg | Calcium: 20mg | Phos: 50mg | Fiber: 2g | Sugar: 4g |

## 6.16   RATATOUILLE AND QUINOA

| PREPARATION TIME | COOKING TIME | SERVING |
|---|---|---|
| 20 mins | 40 mins | 4 |

| INGREDIENTS | DIRECTIONS |
|---|---|
| 1 cup quinoa, uncooked<br>2 cups water<br>1 eggplant, diced<br>2 zucchinis, diced<br>1 red bell pepper, diced<br>1 yellow bell pepper, diced<br>1 onion, chopped<br>2 cloves garlic, minced<br>1 can (14 oz) tomatoes, diced<br>2 tbsp olive oil<br>1 tsp dried basil<br>1 tsp dried thyme | 1. Begin by washing the quinoa and boiling it for 15-20 minutes until it's fully cooked.<br>2. In a pan, heat olive oil over medium-high heat. Add chopped onion and sauté until it becomes translucent.<br>3. Incorporate minced garlic, diced eggplant, diced zucchinis, diced red bell pepper, and diced yellow bell pepper into the pan. Cook for approximately 10 minutes.<br>4. Add canned diced tomatoes (with juice), dried basil, dried thyme, salt, and pepper to the mixture in the pan. Continue cooking for another 10 minutes.<br>5. To serve, layer the herbed quinoa with the ratatouille mixture in a serving bowl. |

**Nutritional facts /value (per serving)**

| Cal: 280 | Carbs: 52g | Protein: 7g | Total Fats: 7g | Sodium: 380mg |
|---|---|---|---|---|
| Pott: 730mg | Calcium: 60mg | Phos: 160mg | Fiber: 9g | Sugar: 9g |

## 6.17   STUFFED MUSHROOMS

| PREPARATION TIME | COOKING TIME | SERVING |
|---|---|---|
| 20 mins | 25 mins | 4 |

| INGREDIENTS | DIRECTIONS |
|---|---|
| 4 large portobello mushrooms, stems removed and gills scraped<br>1 cup cooked quinoa<br>1 cup spinach, chopped<br>½ cup roasted red bell peppers, chopped<br>¼ cup crumbled feta cheese (optional)<br>2 cloves garlic, minced<br>2 tbsp olive oil<br>1 tsp dried oregano | 1. Preheat the oven to 375°F (190°C).<br>2. Take a big bowl and combine cooked quinoa, chopped spinach, chopped roasted red bell peppers, crumbled feta cheese, garlic, olive oil, oregano.<br>3. Stuff each mushroom cap with the quinoa and vegetable mixture.<br>4. Bake in the preheated oven for about 20-25 minutes. |

**Nutritional facts /value (per serving)**

| Cal: 190 | Carbs: 25g | Protein: 6g | Total Fats: 8g | Sodium: 350mg |
|---|---|---|---|---|
| Pott: 660mg | Calcium: 30mg | Phos: 130mg | Fiber: 5g | Sugar: 3g |

## 6.18   KALE RISOTTO AND BUTTERNUT SQUASH

| PREPARATION TIME | COOKING TIME | SERVING |
|---|---|---|
| 15 mins | 30 mins | 4 |

| INGREDIENTS | DIRECTIONS |
|---|---|
| Two tbsp of olive oil<br>1 cup Arborio rice<br>4 cups low-sodium vegetable broth<br>2 cups butternut squash, diced<br>2 cups kale, chopped<br>1 onion, dic<br>2 cloves garlic, crushed<br>Fresh sage leaves, for garnish | 1. Heat vegetable broth over low heat<br>2. Heat olive oil in a pan over medium heat. Add chopped onion and sauté.<br>3. A minced garlic and Arborio rice. Cook for a few minutes<br>4. Start adding the warm vegetable broth one ladle at a time. Allow the liquid to be absorbed before adding more broth. Cook for 20 to 25 minutes.<br>5. In the last minutes of cooking, add diced butternut squash and chopped kale to the pan. Ready to serve. |

**Nutritional facts /value (per serving)**

| Cal: 260 | Carbs: 53g | Protein: 6g | Total Fats: 4g | Sodium: 480mg |
|---|---|---|---|---|
| Pott: 610mg | Calcium: 140mg | Phos: 150mg | Fiber: 4g | Sugar: 3g |

## 6.19   SHRIMP AND ASPARAGUS SKILLET

| PREPARATION TIME | COOKING TIME | SERVING |
|---|---|---|
| 15 mins | 15 mins | 4 |

| INGREDIENTS | DIRECTIONS |
|---|---|
| 1 lb. large shrimp, peeled and deveined<br>1 bunch asparagus, trimmed and cut into 2-inch pieces<br>2 cloves garlic, minced<br>2 tbsp olive oil<br>1 lemon, juice and zest<br>¼ cup chicken broth<br>Salt to taste<br>Black pepper to taste<br>Fresh parsley, for garnish<br>Cooked quinoa, for serving | 1. Sauté minced garlic in olive oil over medium heat<br>2. Add shrimp in it and cook until they turn pink, about 2-3 minutes per side. Remove from the pan and set aside.<br>3. In the same pan, add asparagus pieces and cook for about 5 minutes.<br>4. Add the cooked shrimp to the pan.<br>5. Add chicken broth, lemon zest, and lemon juice. Stir to combine and cook for another minute until heated through.<br>6. Serve the shrimp and asparagus skillet with cooked quinoa. |

### Nutritional facts /value (per serving)

| Cal: 160 | Carbs: 6g | Protein: 20g | Total Fats: 7g | Sodium: 290mg |
|---|---|---|---|---|
| Pott: 330mg | Calcium: 50mg | Phos: 160mg | Fiber: 2g | Sugar: 2g |

## 6.20   SHRIMPS AND SPINACH STIR FRY

| PREPARATION TIME | COOKING TIME | SERVING |
|---|---|---|
| 20 mins | 45 mins | 4 |

| INGREDIENTS | DIRECTIONS |
|---|---|
| 4 oz. shrimps<br>2 cups spinach<br>1-inch piece of ginger, grated<br>¼ cup low-sodium soy sauce or tamari<br>2 tbsp rice vinegar<br>1 tbsp sesame oil<br>1 tsp vegetable oil<br>Sesame seeds and sliced green onions, for garnish | 1. In a pan, add vegetable oil and cook the shrimps for a few minutes until they change color.<br>2. Remove the cooked shrimps from the pan and set them aside. In the same pan, add sesame oil, minced garlic, and grated ginger. Sauté for about a minute until the fragrance emerges.<br>3. Incorporate spinach into the pan and cook for an additional 5 to 7 minutes. Then, reintroduce the cooked shrimps into the pan. |

4. Mix rice vinegar and soy sauce together, and pour this mixture into the pan with the vegetables and tofu.

5. Stir and cook for a few more minutes until everything is thoroughly heated.

### Nutritional facts /value (per serving)

| Cal: 200 | Carbs: 11g | Protein: 15g | Total Fats: 11g | Sodium: 680mg |
|----------|-----------|--------------|-----------------|---------------|
| Pott: 570mg | Calcium: 220mg | Phos: 190mg | Fiber: 4g | Sugar: 3g |

## 6.21   SNOW PEA AND BEEF STIR FRY

| PREPARATION TIME | COOKING TIME | SERVING |
|------------------|--------------|---------|
| 15 mins | 15 mins | 4 |

### INGREDIENTS

1 lb. lean beef (such as sirloin or flank), thinly sliced

2 cups snow peas, trimmed

1 red bell pepper, sliced

1 onion, thinly sliced

2 cloves garlic, minced

2 tbsp low-sodium soy sauce

1 tbsp hoisin sauce

1 tsp sesame oil

1 tbsp vegetable oil

*Sesame seeds, for garnish*

*Cooked brown rice, for serving*

### DIRECTIONS

1. Add vegetable oil in a pan and cook beef slices in it until browned. Remove from the pan and set aside

2. Then in the same pan, add garlic, sliced onion, red bell pepper, and snow peas. Stir-fry for about 3-4 minutes.

3. Add the cooked beef in it

4. Mix soy sauce, hoisin sauce, and sesame oil. Pour this sauce on stir fried mixture and heat it for 2 more minutes.

5. Serve this with cooked rice.

### Nutritional facts /value (per serving)

| Cal: 260 | Carbs: 10g | Protein: 26g | Total Fats: 12g | Sodium: 440mg |
|----------|-----------|--------------|-----------------|---------------|
| Pott: 540mg | Calcium: 30mg | Phos: 270mg | Fiber: 3g | Sugar: 4g |

## 6.22  BEANS AND BROCCOLI STIR FRY

| PREPARATION TIME | COOKING TIME | SERVING |
|---|---|---|
| 15 mins | 15 mins | 4 |

### INGREDIENTS

1 can beans, drained
4 cups broccoli florets
2 cloves garlic, minced
¼ cup low-sodium soy sauce or tamari
2 tbsp hoisin sauce
1 tsp sesame oil
1 tbsp vegetable oil

Sesame seeds and sliced green onions, for garnish
Cooked brown rice or quinoa, for serving

### DIRECTIONS

1. Add vegetable oil in a pan and cook beans for 2 minutes.
2. Then in the same pan, add garlic, broccoli florets. Stir-fry for about 5-7 minutes.
3. Add the cooked beans in it
4. Mix soy sauce, hoisin sauce, and sesame oil. Pour this sauce on stir fried mixture and heat it for 2 more minutes.
5. Serve this with cooked rice.

### Nutritional facts /value (per serving)

| Cal: 230 | Carbs: 10g | Protein: 15g | Total Fats: 15g | Sodium: 680mg |
|---|---|---|---|---|
| Pott: 460mg | Calcium: 100mg | Phos:240mg | Fiber: 3g | Sugar: 3g |

## 6.23  GINGER AND GARLIC CHICKEN STIR-FRY

| PREPARATION TIME | COOKING TIME | SERVING |
|---|---|---|
| 15 mins | 15 mins | 4 |

### INGREDIENTS

1 pound boneless, skinless chicken breast, cut into thin strips
2 tbsp olive oil
2 cloves garlic, minced
1-inch piece of ginger, grated
2 cups broccoli florets
1 red bell pepper, sliced
¼ cup low-sodium soy sauce
1 tbsp honey (or a sugar substitute for a lower-sugar option)
1 tbsp cornstarch (to thicken the sauce)

### DIRECTIONS

1. In a large pan, heat 2 tablespoons of olive oil over medium-high heat.
2. Add minced garlic and grated ginger to the pan, and stir-fry for 1-2 minutes.
3. Incorporate the sliced chicken into the pan and cook until it is no longer pink.
4. Add broccoli and red bell pepper to the pan, and stir-fry until they reach a crisp-tender texture.
5. In a small bowl, whisk together 1/4 cup of low-sodium soy sauce, 1 tablespoon of honey, and 1 tablespoon of cornstarch until you achieve a smooth mixture.
6. Pour the sauce over the chicken and vegetables in the pan, and stir until the sauce thickens.

### Nutritional facts /value (per serving)

| Cal: 300 | Carbs: 25g | Protein: 30g | Total Fats: 12g | Sodium:500mg |
|---|---|---|---|---|
| Pott: 500mg | Calcium: 50mg | Phos: 250mg | Fiber: 4g | Sugar: 6g |

# 7. SNACKS AND SMALL BITES

## 7.1   GRANOLA BAR WITH PEANUT BUTTER

| PREPARATION TIME | COOKING TIME | SERVING |
|---|---|---|
| 20 mins | 15 mins | 5 |

| INGREDIENTS | DIRECTIONS |
|---|---|
| ½ cup old-fashi1d oats, gluten-free<br>¼ cup peanut butter, unsalted, unsweetened, organic<br>2 tbsp chia seeds<br>2 tbsp honey, organic | 6. Preheat the oven to 350F<br>7. Mix old-fashi1d oats, peanut butter, honey, and chia seeds well.<br>8. Take a baking sheet and spread the mixture on it<br>9. Take another sheet and cover the mixture with it.<br>10. Take the rolling pin and press the mixture to spread evenly.<br>11. bake it for 12-15 minutes in the oven.<br>12. When the mixture is baked, take it out and let it cool.<br>13. You can also keep it in the refrigerator for some time.<br>14. Cut into pieces with a sharp knife in your desired shape. |

**Nutritional facts /value (per serving)**

| Cal: 130 | Carbs: 15g | Protein: 6g | Total Fats: 8g | Sodium: 50mg |
|---|---|---|---|---|
| Pott: 170mg | Calcium: 26mg | Phos: 73mg | Fiber: 2 | Sugar: 8g |

## 7.2   NO-BAKE PROTEIN CINNAMON BALLS

| PREPARATION TIME | COOKING TIME | SERVING |
|---|---|---|
| 15 mins | 0 mins | 12 |

| INGREDIENTS | DIRECTIONS |
|---|---|
| 1 cup almond meal<br>1 tsp cinnamon<br>1 cup coconut, shredded<br>2 tbsp butter (it is better to use almond butter)<br>4 tbsp almond milk<br>1 tbsp any whey protein<br>5 dates pitted<br>1 tsp vanilla flavor/extract | 1. Take a blender or food processor.<br>2. Add almond meal, cinnamon, coconut, butter, milk, whey protein, dates, and vanilla flavor.<br>3. Blend and make a smooth paste.<br>4. Now make balls of the mixture.<br>5. Energy balls are ready to use. |

**Nutritional facts /value (per serving)**

| Cal: 170 | Carbs: 14.1g | Protein: 3.2g | Total Fats:10g | Sodium: 5mg |
|---|---|---|---|---|
| Pott: 156mg | Calcium: 2mg | Phos: 33mg | Fiber: 2.6g | Sugar: 9g |

## 7.3    GLUTEN-FREE GINGER ENERGY BALLS

| PREPARATION TIME | COOKING TIME | SERVING |
|---|---|---|
| 15 mins | 0 mins | 12 |

| INGREDIENTS | DIRECTIONS |
|---|---|
| ½ cup old-fashi1d oats, gluten-free<br>¾ cup flaxseed meal, grounded<br>¼ cup coconut, shredded<br>½ tsp ginger, grounded<br>½ tsp cinnamon<br>¼ tsp cloves, grounded<br>¼ tsp salt<br>¼ cup sesame seeds | 1. Combine the almond butter, oats, flaxseed, coconut, sesame seeds, ginger, cloves, cinnamon, and salt in a large mixing bowl.<br>2. Hand-stir the mixture with a spoon until it is well combined and sticky.<br>3. Refrigerate the bowl for 10 minutes so the mixture becomes stiff and easy to form.<br>4. Using wet hands, form 1-inch-sized balls using the dough (squeeze a bit as needed) and lay them on a dish. |

**Nutritional facts /value (per serving)**

| Cal: 100 | Carbs: 7g | Protein: 3.1g | Total Fats: 5g | Sodium: 57mg |
|---|---|---|---|---|
| Pott: 153mg | Calcium: 2.7mg | Phos: 37mg | Fiber: 2.2g | Sugar: 2.8g |

## 7.4    VEGAN SEEDS ENERGY BALLS

| PREPARATION TIME | COOKING TIME | SERVING |
|---|---|---|
| 10-20 mins | 0 mins | 9 |

| INGREDIENTS | DIRECTIONS |
|---|---|
| ½ cup almond flour<br>1/8 cup chia seeds<br>1/8 cup sesame seeds<br>1/8 cup hemp seeds<br>½ cup dates, pitted<br>¼ tsp cinnamon, grounded<br>¼ tsp salt<br>¼ cup sunflower butter | 1. In a food processor, combine all ingredients and process until the dough is sticky and crumbly.<br>2. Take a spoonful of the mixture at a time and press it tightly in your fist before rolling it into a ball form.<br>3. Refrigerate the balls for 10-20 minutes on a tray to firm up.<br>4. Keep in the refrigerator in an airtight BPA-free container. |

**Nutritional facts /value (per serving)**

| Cal: 150 | Carbs: 10.8g | Protein:5.3g | Total Fats: 9.6g | Sodium: 17mg |
|---|---|---|---|---|
| Pott: 164mg | Calcium: 67mg | Phos:121mg | Fiber: 2.1g | Sugar: 5.7g |

## 7.5   *EASY PECAN BARS*

| PREPARATION TIME | COOKING TIME | SERVING |
|---|---|---|
| 35 mins | 6 mins | 15 |

### INGREDIENTS
5 Oz pecans
2 cups old-fashi1d oats
½ cup honey
1 tsp cinnamon, grounded
½ tsp salt
1 cup pecan butter, homemade

### DIRECTIONS
1. Using parchment paper, line a 9-inch square baker.
2. In a skillet, toast the pecans for 4-6 minutes and keep aside.
3. Set aside oats, salt, and cinnamon in a bowl.
4. Add honey and pecan butter in a food processor and blend until making a smooth mixture.
5. Add this liquid mixture to the oats mixture and mix well.
6. Add the chopped pecans and mix again.
7. Pour this mixture into the baker and spread evenly.
8. Refrigerate for 1 hour. After that, cut in the form of medium-sized bars.

### Nutritional facts /value (per serving)

| **Cal:** 220 | **Carbs:** 17.8g | **Protein:**6.3g | **Total Fats:** 16g | **Sodium:** 67mg |
|---|---|---|---|---|
| **Pott:** 184mg | **Calcium:** 96mg | **Phos:**177mg | **Fiber:** 3.1g | **Sugar:** 6.7g |

## 7.6   *NUTTY BERRY ENERGY BALLS*

| PREPARATION TIME | COOKING TIME | SERVING |
|---|---|---|
| 15 mins | 0 mins | 10 |

### INGREDIENTS
1 cup almonds, raw
6 Medjool dates, pitted
½ cup dried berries (Cranberries/Blueberries)
2 tbsp chia seeds
2 tbsp flax seeds
¼ cup coconut flakes, unsweetened
Zest of 1 Lemon
A pinch of salt

### DIRECTIONS
1. Grind the almonds in a food processor until they are gritty.
2. Combine the pitted dates, dried berries, chia seeds, and flax seeds in a food processor
3. Pulse until the mixture comes together.
4. Add the lemon zest and a bit of salt and pulse until thoroughly combined.
5. Form the mixture into balls approximately the size of a golf ball using your palms.
6. Roll the balls in the coconut flakes to evenly coat them.
7. Refrigerate the energy balls for at least 30 minutes.

8. Refrigerate after transferring to an airtight container. Pour this mixture into the baker and spread evenly.
9. Refrigerate for 1 hour. After that, cut in the form of medium-sized bars.

**Nutritional facts /value (per serving)**

| Cal: 120 | Carbs: 16g | Protein: 3g | Total Fats:6g | Sodium: 67mg |
|---|---|---|---|---|
| Pott: 200mg | Calcium: 40mg | Phos: 70mg | Fiber: 4g | Sugar: 10g |

## 7.7

## 7.8    GOOD FAT AVOCADO DIP

| PREPARATION TIME | COOKING TIME | SERVING |
|---|---|---|
| 15 mins | 0 mins | 4 |

| INGREDIENTS | DIRECTIONS |
|---|---|
| 3 Avocados, ripe<br>2 tomatoes, diced<br>½ cup onion, diced<br>1 lime<br>1 tsp salt<br>2 tbsp cilantro, fresh<br>3 garlic cloves, minced | 1. Scoop out the avocado flesh and add it to a bowl.<br>2. Slice through the avocadoes with a knife until they have a chunky consistency.<br>3. Squeeze the lime in the bowl.<br>4. Add tomatoes, onion, cilantro, garlic and salt.<br>5. Mix with the help of a spoon. Ready. |

**Nutritional facts /value (per serving)**

| Cal: 279 | Carbs: 11.8g | Protein:2.3g | Total Fats: 15.9g | Sodium: 307mg |
|---|---|---|---|---|
| Pott: 864mg | Calcium: 36mg | Phos:376mg | Fiber: 8g | Sugar: 1.7g |

## 7.9    VEGAN ARTICHOKE SPINACH DIP

| PREPARATION TIME | COOKING TIME | SERVING |
|---|---|---|
| 10 mins | 15-20 mins | 2 |

| INGREDIENTS | DIRECTIONS |
|---|---|
| 2 cups artichoke hearts<br>2 cups spinach<br>¾ cup milk, nondairy<br>¾ cup raw cashews, unsoaked<br>2 and ½ tbsp lemon juice<br>1 garlic clove<br>1 tsp black pepper<br>1 tsp cayenne pepper | 1. Preheat the oven to 425 degrees Fahrenheit.<br>2. Blender the cashews, lemon juice, milk, garlic, peppers, and salt.<br>3. Blend until completely smooth.<br>4. Mix the artichokes with spinach in the mixture and blend or pulse for a few seconds to integrate them without over-blending to retain a thicker texture.<br>5. Transfer the mixture to an oven-safe baking dish and bake until the top is brown. |

**Nutritional facts /value (per serving)**

| Cal: 359 | Carbs: 25g | Protein: 12g | Total Fats:15g | Sodium: 120mg |
|---|---|---|---|---|
| Pott: 800mg | Calcium: 100mg | Phos: 226mg | Fiber: 8g | Sugar: 5g |

## *7.10  CRISPY ZUCCHINI CHIPS*

| PREPARATION TIME | COOKING TIME | SERVING |
|---|---|---|
| 10 mins | 22 mins | 6 |

| INGREDIENTS | DIRECTIONS |
|---|---|
| 2 zucchinis cut into chips<br>¼ cup all-purpose flour<br>¼ tsp salt<br>¼ tsp garlic powder<br>1 cup breadcrumbs<br>½ cup milk | 1. Preheat the oven to 350F<br>2. Using parchment paper, line a 9-inch baking tray.<br>3. Mix all-purpose flour, milk, salt, and garlic powder in a bowl.<br>4. Add breadcrumbs in a separate small tray.<br>5. Cover the Zucchini first with flour mixture and then breadcrumbs.<br>6. Place the zucchini chips on the baking tray.<br>7. Bake for 20-22 minutes.<br>8. Ready to serve. |

**Nutritional facts /value (per serving)**

| Cal: 279 | Carbs: 11.8g | Protein: 2.3g | Total Fats: 15.9g | Sodium: 307mg |
|---|---|---|---|---|
| Pott: 864mg | Calcium: 36mg | Phos: 376mg | Fiber: 8g | Sugar: 1.7g |

## *7.11  DELICIOUS BEET DIP*

| PREPARATION TIME | COOKING TIME | SERVING |
|---|---|---|
| 20 mins | 40 mins | 8 |

| INGREDIENTS | DIRECTIONS |
|---|---|
| 2 tbsp of olive oil<br>1 and ½ lbs. beets<br>15 Oz chickpeas<br>¼ cup sunflower butter<br>4 garlic cloves<br>1 tsp sea salt<br>1 tsp cumin powder<br>¼ cup lemon juice<br>¼ tsp black pepper | 1. Set the oven to 425 degrees.<br>2. Wash, peel, and cut the beets into ½-inch pieces.<br>3. On a baking sheet lined with foil, toss the beet cubes with salt, black pepper, and oil.<br>4. Lightly oil a small head of garlic and wrap it in foil.<br>5. Place the wrapped garlic on the baking sheet with the beets and bake for 30-40 minutes until the largest beet pieces are fork-soft.<br>6. Allow the beets and garlic to cool.<br>7. Combine the beets, drained chickpeas, garlic, sunflower butter, lemon juice, and |

ground cumin in a food processor.
Process until smooth.

**Nutritional facts /value (per serving)**

| Cal: 189 | Carbs: 21g | Protein: 6g | Total Fats: 9g | Sodium: 320mg |
|---|---|---|---|---|
| Pott: 420mg | Calcium: 60mg | Phos: 140mg | Fiber: 6g | Sugar: 5g |

## 7.12   TWO INGREDIENTS KALE CHIPS

| PREPARATION TIME | COOKING TIME | SERVING |
|---|---|---|
| 5 mins | 10 mins | 2 |

| INGREDIENTS | DIRECTIONS |
|---|---|
| 1 bunch of kale leaves, washed, cleaned<br>1 tbsp virgin olive oil | 1. In a medium mixing bowl, combine kale and olive oil.<br>2. Lay out the greens on a baking sheet.<br>3. Bake the kale for about 10 minutes or until it becomes crispy.<br>4. Ready to serve. |

**Nutritional facts /value (per serving)**

| Cal: 119 | Carbs: 10g | Protein: 4g | Total Fats: 6g | Sodium: 50mg |
|---|---|---|---|---|
| Pott: 600mg | Calcium: 206mg | Phos: 66mg | Fiber: 2g | Sugar: 2g |

## 7.13   BEETROOT CHIPS

| PREPARATION TIME | COOKING TIME | SERVING |
|---|---|---|
| 10 mins | 25-30 mins | 4 |

| INGREDIENTS | DIRECTIONS |
|---|---|
| 4 beetroots, thinly sliced<br>1 tbsp olive oil<br>Sea salt, to taste<br>A pinch of black pepper | 1. Preheat the oven to 180 degrees Celsius (350 degrees Fahrenheit).<br>2. Beets should be washed and peeled. Slice the beets into extremely thin slices<br>3. Toss the beetroot slices in a mixing dish with olive oil, ensuring each piece is well-coated.<br>4. Arrange the slices on a baking tray. To ensure consistent baking, make sure the pieces do not overlap.<br>5. Season the slices gently with sea salt and black pepper.<br>6. Bake for 25-30 minutes or until crispy, keeping an eye on it to prevent scorching. |

**Nutritional facts /value (per serving)**

| Cal: 60 | Carbs: 21g | Protein: 2g | Total Fats: 4g | Sodium: 100mg |
|---|---|---|---|---|
| Pott: 267 mg | Calcium: 22mg | Phos: 42mg | Fiber: 2g | Sugar: 1g |

## 7.14   GARLIC AND LEMON CASHEW DRESSING

| PREPARATION TIME | COOKING TIME | SERVING |
|---|---|---|
| 20 mins | 0 mins | 8 |

| INGREDIENTS | DIRECTIONS |
|---|---|
| 1/3 cup cashews, raw<br>2 tbsp lemon juice<br>½ cup water<br>1 tbsp nutritional yeast<br>1 tbsp capers<br>1 garlic clove, crushed<br>1 tbsp Dijon mustard<br>1 tbsp coconut sugar | 1. In a high-speed blender, combine raw cashews with water.<br>2. Incorporate nutritional yeast, lemon juice, garlic, capers, Dijon mustard, optional coconut sugar, salt, and pepper into the blender.<br>3. Begin blending at a low speed, gradually escalating to high, until the mixture achieves a smooth, creamy texture.<br>4. Taste the dressing and adjust the seasoning with additional lemon juice, garlic, salt, or pepper, adding extra capers or Dijon mustard for a tangier flavor. |

**Nutritional facts /value (per serving)**

| Cal: 50 | Carbs: 4g | Protein: 2g | Total Fats: 3g | Sodium: 75mg |
|---|---|---|---|---|
| Pott: 80mg | Calcium: 10mg | Phos: 40mg | Fiber: 1g | Sugar: 2g |

## 7.15   LIVER FRIENDLY SEEDS MIX

| PREPARATION TIME | COOKING TIME | SERVING |
|---|---|---|
| 5 mins | 10-15 mins | 6 |

| INGREDIENTS | DIRECTIONS |
|---|---|
| ¼ cup sunflower seeds<br>¼ cup walnuts, chopped<br>½ cup almonds, sliced<br>¼ cup chia seeds<br>¼ cup flaxseeds<br>1 tsp turmeric powder | 1. In a mixing dish, combine the seeds and nuts.<br>2. Place them on a parchment-lined baking sheet.<br>3. Mix in the turmeric powder evenly.<br>4. Roast for 10-15 minutes in a preheated oven at 150°C (300°F).<br>5. Allow it to cool before storing it in an airtight container. |

**Nutritional facts /value (per serving)**

| Cal: 150 | Carbs: 7g | Protein: 6g | Total Fats:11g | Sodium: 5mg |
|---|---|---|---|---|
| Pott: 180mg | Calcium: 60mg | Phos: 120mg | Fiber: 4g | Sugar: 0g |

## 7.16   SEED AND NUT BUTTER

| PREPARATION TIME | COOKING TIME | SERVING |
|---|---|---|
| 10 mins | 0 mins | 8 |

| INGREDIENTS | DIRECTIONS |
|---|---|
| ½ cup almonds<br>½ cup cashews<br>2 tbsp flaxseeds<br>1 tbsp coconut oil<br>½ tsp salt | 1. Combine the cashews, flaxseeds, and almonds in a food processor.<br>2. Finely grind until smooth.<br>3. Mix in the coconut oil and season with salt.<br>4. Continue to process until the mixture is smooth and creamy.<br>5. Keep in an airtight container. |

**Nutritional facts /value (per serving)**

| Cal: 180 | Carbs: 8g | Protein: 6g | Total Fats: 15g | Sodium: 50mg |
|---|---|---|---|---|
| Pott: 210mg | Calcium: 60mg | Phos: 120mg | Fiber: 3g | Sugar: 2g |

## 7.17   CHIA SEED AND ALMOND DRINK

| PREPARATION TIME | COOKING TIME | SERVING |
|---|---|---|
| 15 mins | 0 mins | 2 |

| INGREDIENTS | DIRECTIONS |
|---|---|
| 1 cup almond milk<br>1 tbsp chia seeds<br>1 tbsp almond butter<br>½ small banana<br>½ tsp cinnamon powder<br>Ice | 1. Blend chia seeds, almond milk, almond butter, and cinnamon in a blender.<br>2. Blend until the mixture is smooth and creamy.<br>3. Blend in the ice cubes until well cold.<br>4. Serve in a glass right away. |

**Nutritional facts /value (per serving)**

| Cal: 200 | Carbs: 18g | Protein: 6g | Total Fats: 12g | Sodium: 80mg |
|---|---|---|---|---|
| Pott: 300mg | Calcium: 150mg | Phos:100mg | Fiber: 6g | Sugar: 9g |

## 7.18   SEED CRACKERS

| PREPARATION TIME | COOKING TIME | SERVING |
|---|---|---|
| 30 mins | 20-25 mins | 10 |

| INGREDIENTS | DIRECTIONS |
|---|---|
| ½ cup flaxseeds<br>¼ cup sesame seeds<br>¼ cup sunflower seeds<br>¼ cup pumpkin seeds<br>1 cup water<br>1 tsp garlic powder<br>1 tsp onion powder | 1. Set your oven's temperature to 350 °F (175 °C).<br>2. Add water, garlic powder, onion powder, sea salt, sesame, sunflower, pumpkin, and flaxseeds to a bowl. The flaxseeds will gel if you let it sit for 15-20 minutes. |

½ tsp sea salt

3. On a baking pan with parchment paper coated, thinly spread the mixture.
4. Once brown and crispy, bake for 20 to 25 minutes, splitting them halfway through.
5. Before breaking them into separate crackers, let them cool.

**Nutritional facts /value (per serving)**

| Cal: 100 | Carbs: 5g | Protein: 4g | Total Fats: 8g | Sodium: 200mg |
|---|---|---|---|---|
| Pott: 150mg | Calcium: 70mg | Phos: 150mg | Fiber: 4g | Sugar: 0g |

## 7.19   ROASTED SPICED PUMPKIN SEEDS

| PREPARATION TIME | COOKING TIME | SERVING |
|---|---|---|
| 10 mins | 20-30 mins | 4 |

| INGREDIENTS | DIRECTIONS |
|---|---|
| 2 cups raw pumpkin seeds, washed and dried<br>1 tbsp olive oil<br>1 tsp smoked paprika<br>½ tsp turmeric<br>½ tsp garlic powder<br>Salt to taste | 1. Set your oven's temperature to 350 °F (175 °C).<br>2. Combine the pumpkin seeds, olive oil, garlic powder, smoked paprika, turmeric, and salt in a mixing bowl. Mix vigorously until the spices and oil are uniformly distributed throughout the seeds.<br>3. Line a baking sheet with parchment paper and distribute the seeds evenly.<br>4. Bake for 25-30 minutes, stirring halfway during cooking time, or until the seeds are brown and crispy.<br>5. Remove from the oven and cool fully. |

**Nutritional facts /value (per serving)**

| Cal: 200 | Carbs: 4g | Protein: 9g | Total Fats: 18g | Sodium: 200mg |
|---|---|---|---|---|
| Pott: 226mg | Calcium: 12mg | Phos:397mg | Fiber: 2g | Sugar: 0g |

## 7.20   COLORFUL FRUIT MIX

| PREPARATION TIME | COOKING TIME | SERVING |
|---|---|---|
| 20 mins | 0 mins | 4 |

| INGREDIENTS | DIRECTIONS |
|---|---|
| 2 apples, diced<br>1 cup blueberries<br>1 banana, sliced<br>1 orange, peeled and segmented<br>1 tbsp chia seeds<br>1 tbsp flax seeds<br>1 tbsp lemon juice<br>1 tbsp mint leaves, chopped | 1. Combine the chopped apples, blueberries, banana slices, and orange segments in a large mixing dish.<br>2. Chia and flax seeds, recognized for their ability to support liver function, should be added to the combination. |

1 tsp cinnamon, ground

3. Lemon juice should be drizzled on top to give the meal a fresh zing and stop the fruit from browning.
4. Toss everything together until thoroughly blended, then add the minced mint leaves and ground cinnamon.

**Nutritional facts /value (per serving)**

| **Cal:** 120 | **Carbs:** 27g | **Protein:** 6g | **Total Fats:** 1.5g | **Sodium:** 3mg |
|---|---|---|---|---|
| **Pott:** 260mg | **Calcium:** 50mg | **Phos:** 40mg | **Fiber:** 6g | **Sugar:** 14g |

## 7.21   KIWI AND BERRY BLISS

| PREPARATION TIME | COOKING TIME | SERVING |
|---|---|---|
| 10 mins | 0 mins | 2 |

| INGREDIENTS | DIRECTIONS |
|---|---|
| 2 kiwis, peeled and sliced<br>1 cup mixed berries (strawberries, blueberries, raspberries)<br>1 tbsp chia seeds<br>a handful of mint leaves, finely chopped<br>1 tbsp lemon juice | 1. Combine the cut kiwis and mixed berries in a mixing dish.<br>2. Drizzle the lemon juice over the fruit and gently toss to incorporate.<br>3. Chia seeds may be sprinkled over the fruits to provide crunch and nutrients.<br>4. If you want to add a touch of sweetness, garnish with fresh mint leaves.<br>5. Serve immediately as a light snack. |

**Nutritional facts /value (per serving)**

| **Cal:** 90 | **Carbs:** 20g | **Protein:** 2g | **Total Fats:** 1g | **Sodium:** 5g |
|---|---|---|---|---|
| **Pott:** 350mg | **Calcium:** 50mg | **Phos:** 60mg | **Fiber:** 5g | **Sugar:** 9g |

## 7.22   CITRUS FRUIT MIX

| PREPARATION TIME | COOKING TIME | SERVING |
|---|---|---|
| 10 mins | 0 mins | 2 |

| INGREDIENTS | DIRECTIONS |
|---|---|
| 1 grapefruit, segmented<br>2 oranges, segmented<br>2 kiwis, sliced<br>1 handful of fresh mint leaves, chopped<br>1 tbsp chia seeds - | 1. Combine grapefruit and orange segments in a mixing dish.<br>2. Mix carefully after adding the chopped kiwi.<br>3. Before serving, sprinkle with fresh mint and chia seeds. |

**Nutritional facts /value (per serving)**

| **Cal:** 130 | **Carbs:** 27g | **Protein:** 3g | **Total Fats:** 2g | **Sodium:** 2mg |
|---|---|---|---|---|
| **Pott:** 450mg | **Calcium:** 70mg | **Phos:** 60mg | **Fiber:** 6g | **Sugar:** 8g |

## 7.23 TROPICAL PAPAYA & PINEAPPLE COMBO

| PREPARATION TIME | COOKING TIME | SERVING |
|---|---|---|
| 15 mins | 0 mins | 2 |

| INGREDIENTS | DIRECTIONS |
|---|---|
| 1 medium papaya, peeled and diced<br>1 cup pineapple, diced<br>1 mango, peeled and diced<br>2 tbsp coconut flakes<br>1 tsp lime zest<br>2 tbsp fresh lime juice | 1. Combine the chopped papaya, pineapple, and mango in a large mixing basin.<br>2. Garnish with lime zest and sprinkle with fresh lime juice. Gently toss to mix.<br>3. Garnish with coconut flakes if desired.<br>4. Serve chilled as a light and nutritious salad. |

### Nutritional facts /value (per serving)

| Cal: 140 | Carbs: 31g | Protein: 2g | Total Fats: 2g | Sodium: 3mg |
|---|---|---|---|---|
| Pott: 500mg | Calcium: 40mg | Phos: 50mg | Fiber: 5g | Sugar: 11g |

## 7.24 BERRY & MELON MEDLEY

| PREPARATION TIME | COOKING TIME | SERVING |
|---|---|---|
| 10 mins | 0 mins | 2 |

| INGREDIENTS | DIRECTIONS |
|---|---|
| 1 cup watermelon, cubed<br>1 cup cantaloupe, cubed<br>½ cup blueberries<br>½ cup blackberries<br>½ cup Greek yogurt (for serving)<br>1 tbsp honey (optional)<br>A handful of fresh basil leaves, chopped | 1. Combine the diced watermelon and cantaloupe in a mixing basin.<br>2. Toss the blueberries and blackberries into the basin to combine.<br>3. If preferred, serve the fruit mixture with a side of Greek yogurt drizzled with honey.<br>4. Garnish with fresh basil leaves for a unique and refreshing flavor combination.<br>5. Serve as a healthy snack. |

### Nutritional facts /value (per serving)

| Cal: 130 | Carbs: 28g | Protein: 5g | Total Fats: 1g | Sodium: 30mg |
|---|---|---|---|---|
| Pott: 400mg | Calcium: 100mg | Phos: 50mg | Fiber: 4g | Sugar: 8g |

## 7.25   APPLE & WALNUT CRUNCH MIX

| PREPARATION TIME | COOKING TIME | SERVING |
|---|---|---|
| 10 mins | 0 mins | 2 |

### INGREDIENTS

2 medium apples, chopped
¼ cup walnuts, chopped
½ tsp cinnamon
½ cup Greek yogurt (low-fat)
Fresh mint leaves for garnish

### DIRECTIONS

1. Combine the chopped apples and walnuts in a mixing basin.
2. Sprinkle cinnamon on top and blend thoroughly.
3. Divide the mixture into 2 portions and top with a dollop of Greek yogurt on top of each.
4. Garnish with fresh mint leaves if desired.
5. Enjoy your nutritious, crispy snack

### Nutritional facts /value (per serving)

| Cal: 150 | Carbs: 20g | Protein: 5g | Total Fats: 7g | Sodium: 3mg |
|---|---|---|---|---|
| Pott: 200mg | Calcium: 60mg | Phos: 65mg | Fiber: 4g | Sugar: 5g |

# 8. LIVER-CLEANSING JUICES AND SMOOTHIES

## 8.1 CUCUMBER MINT BLISS

| PREPARATION TIME | COOKING TIME | SERVING |
|---|---|---|
| 10 mins | 0 mins | 2 |

| INGREDIENTS | DIRECTIONS |
|---|---|
| 1 cucumber, sliced<br>1 small green apple, sliced<br>1 cup spinach leaves<br>A handful of fresh mint leaves<br>1 lime, juiced<br>1 cup coconut water<br>1 tbsp chia seeds | 1. In a blender, combine all the ingredients.<br>2. Blend till creamy and smooth.<br>3. Serve cold glasses right away. |

### Nutritional facts /value (per serving)

| Cal: 95 | Carbs: 18g | Protein: 2g | Total Fats: 2g | Sodium: 55mg |
|---|---|---|---|---|
| Pott: 410mg | Calcium: 60mg | Phos: 50mg | Fiber: 5g | Sugar: 10g |

## 8.2 GINGER SPINACH GREENIE

| PREPARATION TIME | COOKING TIME | SERVING |
|---|---|---|
| 10 mins | 0 mins | 1 |

| INGREDIENTS | DIRECTIONS |
|---|---|
| 1 banana<br>1 cup spinach leaves<br>½ inch ginger, grated<br>1 cup almond milk, unsweetened<br>½ lemon, juiced<br>1 tbsp flaxseeds | 1. In a blender, combine all the ingredients.<br>2. Blend till creamy and smooth.<br>3. Serve cold glasses right away. |

### Nutritional facts /value (per serving)

| Cal: 145 | Carbs: 25g | Protein: 4g | Total Fats: 4g | Sodium: 80mg |
|---|---|---|---|---|
| Pott: 490mg | Calcium: 200mg | Phos: 70mg | Fiber: 6g | Sugar: 12g |

## 8.3 KALE PINEAPPLE DELIGHT

| PREPARATION TIME | COOKING TIME | SERVING |
|---|---|---|
| 10 mins | 0 mins | 3 |

| INGREDIENTS | DIRECTIONS |
|---|---|
| 1 cup kale, chopped<br>½ cup pineapple chunks<br>1 green apple, cored and sliced<br>1 orange, peeled<br>1 cup coconut water<br>1 tbsp hemp seeds | 1. Combine kale, pineapple, green apple, and orange in a blender.<br>2. Blend until smooth after adding the coconut water.<br>3. Add the hemp seeds, then mix for a short while more. |

**Nutritional facts /value (per serving)**

| Cal: 110 | Carbs: 23g | Protein: 3g | Total Fats: 2g | Sodium: 50mg |
|---|---|---|---|---|
| Pott: 430mg | Calcium: 70mg | Phos: 60mg | Fiber: 4g | Sugar: 17g |

## 8.4 REFRESHING AVOCADO GREEN SMOOTHIE

| PREPARATION TIME | COOKING TIME | SERVING |
|---|---|---|
| 10 mins | 0 mins | 4 |

| INGREDIENTS | DIRECTIONS |
|---|---|
| 1 avocado, peeled and pitted<br>1 cup spinach leaves<br>1 cucumber, sliced<br>1 lime, juiced<br>1 ½ cup water<br>A handful of fresh mint leaves<br>2 tbsp honey | 1. In a blender, combine avocado, spinach, cucumber, lime juice, and water.<br>2. Add honey and mint leaves.<br>3. Blend till creamy and smooth.<br>4. Ready to serve |

**Nutritional facts /value (per serving)**

| Cal: 140 | Carbs: 18g | Protein: 2g | Total Fats: 8g | Sodium: 30mg |
|---|---|---|---|---|
| Pott: 520mg | Calcium: 40mg | Phos: 55mg | Fiber: 6g | Sugar: 12g |

## 8.5 GINGER LEMON DETOX SMOOTHIE

| PREPARATION TIME | COOKING TIME | SERVING |
|---|---|---|
| 10 mins | 0 mins | 1 |

| INGREDIENTS | DIRECTIONS |
|---|---|
| 1 green apple, cored and sliced<br>1 lemon, juiced<br>1 small piece of fresh ginger, peeled<br>1 cup spinach leaves<br>½ cup water<br>1 tsp chia seeds | 1. Blend the green apple slices, lemon juice, and fresh ginger in a blender.<br>2. Blend spinach greens and water till smooth.<br>3. Blend briefly to mix the chia seeds.<br>4. Serve in a glass right away. |

**Nutritional facts /value (per serving)**

| Cal: 90 | Carbs: 21g | Protein: 2g | Total Fats: 1g | Sodium: 20mg |
|---|---|---|---|---|
| Pott: 340mg | Calcium: 50mg | Phos: 40mg | Fiber: 5g | Sugar: 14g |

## 8.6 SPIRULINA & MINT GREEN SMOOTHIE

| PREPARATION TIME | COOKING TIME | SERVING |
|---|---|---|
| 10 mins | 0 mins | 1 |

| INGREDIENTS | DIRECTIONS |
|---|---|
| 1 banana<br>1 tsp spirulina powder<br>A handful of fresh mint leaves<br>½ cucumber, sliced<br>1 cup coconut water<br>1 tbsp chia seeds | 1. Take a blender.<br>2. In the blender, add the banana, spirulina powder, fresh mint leaves, and sliced cucumber.<br>3. Blend in the coconut water until the mixture is smooth and creamy.<br>4. Allow the chia seeds to settle for a few minutes to thicken.<br>5. Pour into a glass and serve. |

**Nutritional facts /value (per serving)**

| Cal: 170 | Carbs: 40g | Protein: 4g | Total Fats: 2g | Sodium: 70mg |
|---|---|---|---|---|
| Pott: 600mg | Calcium: 100mg | Phos: 90mg | Fiber: 10g | Sugar: 18g |

## 8.7 TRIPLE BERRY BLISS

| PREPARATION TIME | COOKING TIME | SERVING |
|---|---|---|
| 10 mins | 0 mins | 6 |

| INGREDIENTS | DIRECTIONS |
|---|---|
| 3 cups strawberries, halved<br>½ cups blueberries<br>½ cups raspberries<br>3 bananas<br>3 cups almond milk<br>2 tbsp of chia seeds | 1. In a blender, combine strawberries, blueberries, raspberries, and bananas.<br>2. Blend in the almond milk until smooth.<br>3. Stir in chia seeds for an added nutrient boost.<br>4. Serve in glasses and enjoy right away. |

**Nutritional facts /value (per serving)**

| Cal: 150 | Carbs: 30g | Protein: 4g | Total Fats: 3g | Sodium: 50mg |
|---|---|---|---|---|
| Pott: 500mg | Calcium: 200mg | Phos: 100mg | Fiber: 7g | Sugar: 18g |

## 8.8 BERRY MANGO FUSION

| PREPARATION TIME | COOKING TIME | SERVING |
|---|---|---|
| 10 mins | 0 mins | 8 |

| INGREDIENTS | DIRECTIONS |
|---|---|
| 4 cups mixed berries (strawberries, blueberries, raspberries)<br>2 ripe mangos, peeled and pitted<br>4 cups coconut water<br>2 tbsp ground flaxseeds<br>A handful of fresh mint leaves | 1. In a blender, combine the mixed berries and mango pieces.<br>2. Add coconut water and blend until smooth and creamy.<br>3. Stir in the ground flaxseeds for a nutritious boost. |

4. Serve in individual cups, garnished with a mint leaf.

## Nutritional facts /value (per serving)

| Cal: 135 | Carbs: 30g | Protein: 2g | Total Fats: 1g | Sodium: 40mg |
|---|---|---|---|---|
| Pott: 420mg | Calcium: 50mg | Phos: 60mg | Fiber: 5g | Sugar: 14g |

# 8.9 MIXED BERRY AND SPINACH DELIGHT

| PREPARATION TIME | COOKING TIME | SERVING |
|---|---|---|
| 15 mins | 0 mins | 6 |

| INGREDIENTS | DIRECTIONS |
|---|---|
| 3 cups mixed berries (strawberries, blueberries, blackberries)<br>2 cups fresh spinach<br>2 cups Greek yogurt<br>2 tbsp honey<br>A pinch of ground cinnamon | 1. In a blender, combine mixed berries and fresh spinach.<br>2. Add Greek yogurt, honey, and a pinch of ground cinnamon.<br>3. Blend until smooth and creamy.<br>4. Serve in individual cups. |

## Nutritional facts /value (per serving)

| Cal: 120 | Carbs: 22g | Protein: 5g | Total Fats: 1g | Sodium: 35mg |
|---|---|---|---|---|
| Pott: 300mg | Calcium: 100mg | Phos: 80mg | Fiber: 4g | Sugar: 16g |

# 8.10 EXOTIC BERRY AND KIWI BLEND

| PREPARATION TIME | COOKING TIME | SERVING |
|---|---|---|
| 10 mins | 0 mins | 8 |

| INGREDIENTS | DIRECTIONS |
|---|---|
| 4 cups mixed berries (strawberries, raspberries, blueberries)<br>4 kiwis, peeled and sliced<br>4 cups coconut water<br>2 tbsp of chia seeds | 1. Combine mixed berries and sliced kiwis in a blender.<br>2. Add coconut water and blend until smooth.<br>3. Stir in chia seeds for an extra nutrient punch.<br>4. Serve in glasses, enjoy this exotic blend as a rejuvenating morning drink or snack. |

## Nutritional facts /value (per serving)

| Cal: 130 | Carbs: 30g | Protein: 3g | Total Fats: 2g | Sodium: 44mg |
|---|---|---|---|---|
| Pott: 430mg | Calcium: 60mg | Phos: 90mg | Fiber: 5g | Sugar: 20g |

## 8.11 BERRY AND OAT SMOOTHIE

| PREPARATION TIME | COOKING TIME | SERVING |
|---|---|---|
| 12 mins | 0 mins | 6 |

| INGREDIENTS | DIRECTIONS |
|---|---|
| 3 cups mixed berries (blueberries, raspberries, blackberries)<br>½ cups rolled oats<br>3 cups almond milk<br>2 tbsp flaxseeds<br>1 tbsp honey (optional)<br>1 tsp vanilla extract | 1. In a blender, add the mixed berries and almond milk. Blend until smooth.<br>2. Incorporate the rolled oats, flaxseeds, honey, and vanilla extract. Blend until well combined.<br>3. Serve in individual cups topped with a few fresh berries and a sprinkle of oats.<br>4. Enjoy this hearty smoothie. |

**Nutritional facts /value (per serving)**

| Cal: 150 | Carbs: 28g | Protein: 5g | Total Fats: 3g | Sodium: 60mg |
|---|---|---|---|---|
| Pott: 300mg | Calcium: 120mg | Phos: 110mg | Fiber: 6g | Sugar: 10g |

## 8.12 BERRY AND NUT BLEND

| PREPARATION TIME | COOKING TIME | SERVING |
|---|---|---|
| 10 mins | 0 mins | 8 |

| INGREDIENTS | DIRECTIONS |
|---|---|
| 4 cups mixed berries (strawberries, blueberries, cranberries)<br>2 bananas, sliced<br>2 cups Greek yogurt<br>1 cup mixed nuts (almonds, walnuts), slightly chopped<br>2 tbsp honey<br>1 tbsp ground cinnamon | 1. In a blender, add the mixed berries and sliced bananas. Blend until smooth.<br>2. Stir in Greek yogurt, honey, and ground cinnamon until well combined.<br>3. Serve in individual cups topped with a sprinkling of mixed nuts. |

**Nutritional facts /value (per serving)**

| Cal: 180 | Carbs: 25g | Protein: 7g | Total Fats: 8g | Sodium: 66mg |
|---|---|---|---|---|
| Pott: 350mg | Calcium: 130mg | Phos: 150mg | Fiber: 5g | Sugar: 18g |

## 8.13 TURMERIC AND GINGER INFUSION

| PREPARATION TIME | COOKING TIME | SERVING |
|---|---|---|
| 10 mins | 5 mins | 6 |

| INGREDIENTS | DIRECTIONS |
|---|---|
| 6 cups water<br>1 tbsp fresh ginger, grated<br>1 tbsp fresh turmeric, grated<br>1 lemon, juiced<br>2 tbsp honey (optional) | 1. In a pot, bring water to a boil.<br>2. Add the grated ginger and turmeric. Let it simmer for 5 minutes.<br>3. Turn off the heat and stir in the lemon juice and honey. |

Fresh mint leaves (for garnish)

4. Strain the infusion into cups, garnish with fresh mint leaves, and serve.

**Nutritional facts /value (per serving)**

| Cal: 30 | Carbs: 6g | Protein: 0g | Total Fats: 0g | Sodium: 10mg |
|---|---|---|---|---|
| Pott: 50mg | Calcium:20mg | Phos: 15mg | Fiber: 0g | Sugar: 5g |

## 8.14 BEET AND LEMON DETOX JUICE

| PREPARATION TIME | COOKING TIME | SERVING |
|---|---|---|
| 15 mins | 0 mins | 8 |

| INGREDIENTS | DIRECTIONS |
|---|---|
| 4 beets, peeled and quartered<br>2 carrots, chopped<br>1 lemon, juiced<br>1 apple, cored and chopped<br>1 tbsp ginger, grated<br>1 cucumber, chopped | 1. In a juicer, add beets, carrots, apple, and cucumber to extract the juice.<br>2. Stir in the lemon juice and grated ginger.<br>3. Serve in individual cups and enjoy this refreshing detox juice as a morning or afternoon treat. |

**Nutritional facts /value (per serving)**

| Cal: 60 | Carbs: 14g | Protein: 1g | Total Fats: 0g | Sodium: 40mg |
|---|---|---|---|---|
| Pott: 300mg | Calcium: 25mg | Phos: 40mg | Fiber: 3g | Sugar: 10g |

## 8.15 GREEN TEA AND LEMON INFUSION

| PREPARATION TIME | COOKING TIME | SERVING |
|---|---|---|
| 5 mins | 5 mins | 6 |

| INGREDIENTS | DIRECTIONS |
|---|---|
| 6 green tea bags<br>6 cups water<br>1 lemon, sliced<br>1 tbsp honey (optional)<br>Fresh mint leaves (for garnish) | 1. Boil the water in a large pot.<br>2. Once boiling, turn off the heat and add the green tea bags. Let it steep for 3-4 minutes.<br>3. Remove the tea bags and add the lemon slices and honey, if using.<br>4. Stir well and garnish with fresh mint leaves before serving. |

**Nutritional facts /value (per serving)**

| Cal: 10 | Carbs: 2g | Protein: 0g | Total Fats: 0g | Sodium: 5mg |
|---|---|---|---|---|
| Pott: 30mg | Calcium: 10mg | Phos: 5mg | Fiber: 0 | Sugar: 2g |

## 8.16 SPIRULINA AND PINEAPPLE SMOOTHIE

| PREPARATION TIME | COOKING TIME | SERVING |
|---|---|---|
| 10 mins | 0 mins | 8 |

| INGREDIENTS | DIRECTIONS |
|---|---|
| 2 cups pineapple, cubed<br>1 banana<br>2 tbsp spirulina powder<br>2 cups spinach leaves<br>2 cups coconut water<br>1 tbsp honey (optional) | 1. Combine pineapple, banana, spirulina powder, and spinach leaves in a blender.<br>2. Pour in coconut water and blend until smooth.<br>3. Taste and add honey if needed for sweetness.<br>4. Serve chilled in individual cups, garnished with a small pineapple slice. |

Nutritional facts /value (per serving)

| Cal: 85 | Carbs: 19g | Protein: 2g | Total Fats: 0g | Sodium: 55mg |
|---|---|---|---|---|
| Pott: 410mg | Calcium: 45mg | Phos: 30mg | Fiber: 3g | Sugar: 14g |

## 8.17 DANDELION GREEN SMOOTHIE

| PREPARATION TIME | COOKING TIME | SERVING |
|---|---|---|
| 10 mins | 0 mins | 6 |

| INGREDIENTS | DIRECTIONS |
|---|---|
| 2 cups dandelion greens, washed and chopped<br>2 green apples, chopped<br>1 lemon, juiced<br>1tsp ginger, peeled and grated<br>6 cups water | 1. Combine all the ingredients in a blender.<br>2. Blend until smooth and creamy.<br>3. Serve immediately, garnished with a slice of lemon if desired. |

Nutritional facts /value (per serving)

| Cal: 50 | Carbs: 12g | Protein: 1g | Total Fats: 0g | Sodium: 10mg |
|---|---|---|---|---|
| Pott: 200mg | Calcium: 50mg | Phos: 30mg | Fiber: 3g | Sugar: 8g |

## 8.18 MILK THISTLE AND BLUEBERRY SMOOTHIE

| PREPARATION TIME | COOKING TIME | SERVING |
|---|---|---|
| 10 mins | 0 mins | 6 |

| INGREDIENTS | DIRECTIONS |
|---|---|
| 1 tbsp milk thistle seeds<br>2 cups blueberries<br>1 banana<br>1 tbsp chia seeds<br>6 cups almond milk | 1. Blend the milk thistle seeds until they turn into a fine powder.<br>2. Add the blueberries, banana, chia seeds, and almond milk.<br>3. Blend until smooth. |

Nutritional facts /value (per serving)

| Cal: 100 | Carbs: 16g | Protein: 2g | Total Fats: 3g | Sodium: 100mg |
|---|---|---|---|---|
| Pott: 250mg | Calcium: 200mg | Phos: 100mg | Fiber: 4g | Sugar: 10g |

## 8.19 TOMATO & RED BELL PEPPER BLEND

| PREPARATION TIME | COOKING TIME | SERVING |
| --- | --- | --- |
| 10 mins | 0 mins | 8 |

| INGREDIENTS | DIRECTIONS |
| --- | --- |
| 4 large tomatoes, chopped<br>2 red bell peppers, seeds removed and chopped<br>1 small red onion, peeled and chopped<br>1 lemon, juiced<br>A pinch of black pepper<br>2 cups cold water | 1. Add tomatoes, red bell peppers, and red onion to a blender or juicer.<br>2. Include lemon juice, black pepper, and water.<br>3. Blend or juice until smooth, adding more water if necessary.<br>4. Serve chilled, sprinkled with a touch of black pepper on top. |

**Nutritional facts /value (per serving)**

| Cal: 40 | Carbs: 9g | Protein: 1.5g | Total Fats: 0.2g | Sodium: 20mg |
| --- | --- | --- | --- | --- |
| Pott: 280mg | Calcium: 15mg | Phos: 25mg | Fiber: 2g | Sugar: 6g |

## 8.20 APPLE & CARROT JUICE

| PREPARATION TIME | COOKING TIME | SERVING |
| --- | --- | --- |
| 15 mins | 0 mins | 6 |

| INGREDIENTS | DIRECTIONS |
| --- | --- |
| 3 carrots, peeled and chopped<br>1 apple, cored and chopped<br>1 inch of fresh ginger, peeled<br>2 cups cold water | 1. Combine carrots, apple, and ginger in a juicer or blender.<br>2. Add water and blend or juice until smooth.<br>3. If using a blender, strain the mixture to remove the pulp.<br>4. Serve chilled, enjoy this sweet and savory blend. |

**Nutritional facts /value (per serving)**

| Cal: 70 | Carbs: 16g | Protein: 1g | Total Fats: 0.3g | Sodium: 45mg |
| --- | --- | --- | --- | --- |
| Pott: 330mg | Calcium: 30mg | Phos: 35mg | Fiber: 3g | Sugar: 9g |

## 8.21 BEETS & GINGER JUICE

| PREPARATION TIME | COOKING TIME | SERVING |
| --- | --- | --- |
| 10 mins | 0 mins | 6 |

| INGREDIENTS | DIRECTIONS |
| --- | --- |
| 3 medium beets, peeled and chopped<br>2 apples, cored and chopped<br>1 inch of fresh ginger, peeled<br>1 lemon, juiced<br>2 cups cold water | 1. Combine beets, apples, and ginger in a juicer or blender.<br>2. Add lemon juice and water. |

3. Blend or juice until smooth. If using a blender, strain the mixture to remove the pulp.
4. Serve chilled.

**Nutritional facts /value (per serving)**

| Cal: 65 | Carbs: 15g | Protein: 1g | Total Fats: 0.2g | Sodium: 40mg |
|---------|------------|-------------|------------------|--------------|
| Pott: 320mg | Calcium: 20mg | Phos: 30mg | Fiber: 3g | Sugar: 12g |

## 8.22 COOL CUCUMBER & CELERY COMBO

| PREPARATION TIME | COOKING TIME | SERVING |
|------------------|--------------|---------|
| 10 mins | 0 mins | 8 |

| INGREDIENTS | DIRECTIONS |
|-------------|------------|
| 4 cucumbers, sliced<br>4 celery stalks, chopped<br>1 green apple, cored and chopped<br>1 handful of fresh mint leaves<br>1 lime, juiced<br>2 cups cold water | 1. In a blender or juicer, add cucumbers, celery stalks, and green apple.<br>2. Add mint leaves, lime juice, and water.<br>3. Blend or juice until smooth, adding more water if necessary.<br>4. Strain the juice to remove the pulp, if preferred.<br>5. Serve chilled for a refreshing and nourishing drink. |

**Nutritional facts /value (per serving)**

| Cal: 45 | Carbs: 11g | Protein: 1.5g | Total Fats: 0.2g | Sodium: 35mg |
|---------|------------|---------------|------------------|--------------|
| Pott: 280mg | Calcium: 35mg | Phos: 20mg | Fiber: 2g | Sugar: 7g |

## 8.23 GREEN VEGGIES JUICE

| PREPARATION TIME | COOKING TIME | SERVING |
|------------------|--------------|---------|
| 10 mins | 0 mins | 6 |

| INGREDIENTS | DIRECTIONS |
|-------------|------------|
| 4 cups kale leaves, washed and torn<br>2 cucumbers, sliced<br>4 celery stalks, chopped<br>1 lemon, peeled<br>1-inch fresh turmeric root, peeled<br>2 inches fresh ginger root, peeled<br>1 tbsp milk thistle seeds | 1. Prepare all the vegetables, making sure to clean them thoroughly.<br>2. Grind the milk thistle seeds to a fine powder.<br>3. In a juicer, juice the kale, cucumbers, celery, lemon, turmeric, and ginger.<br>4. Stir in the milk thistle powder and mix well. |

**Nutritional facts /value (per serving)**

| Cal: 55 | Carbs: 12g | Protein: 3g | Total Fats: 0.5g | Sodium: 30mg |
|---------|------------|-------------|------------------|--------------|
| Pott: 400mg | Calcium: 100mg | Phos: 40mg | Fiber: 3g | Sugar: 5mog |

## 8.24 RADIANT RED DETOX

| PREPARATION TIME | COOKING TIME | SERVING |
|---|---|---|
| 10 mins | 0 mins | 6 |

### INGREDIENTS
3 medium-sized beets, peeled and chopped
3 carrots, peeled and chopped
1 red bell pepper, deseeded and sliced
1 small red cabbage, chopped
1 lemon, peeled
1 tbsp hemp seeds

### DIRECTIONS
1. Prepare your vegetables by washing and chopping them.
2. In a juicer, process the beets, carrots, bell pepper, cabbage, and lemon.
3. Grind the hemp seeds into a fine powder and stir into the juice.
4. Serve immediately to enjoy a vibrant, nutrient-dense juice

### Nutritional facts /value (per serving)

| Cal: 70 | Carbs: 16g | Protein: 3g | Total Fats: 1g | Sodium: 40mg |
|---|---|---|---|---|
| Pott: 450mg | Calcium: 60mg | Phos: 50mg | Fiber: 4g | Sugar: 10g |

# 9. FRUIT-BASED DESSERTS

## 9.1  MANGO SORBET

| PREPARATION TIME | FREEZING TIME | SERVING |
|---|---|---|
| 10 mins | 4 hrs. | 4 |

| INGREDIENTS | DIRECTIONS |
|---|---|
| 4 cups frozen mango chunks<br>2 tbsp lemon juice<br>1 tbsp honey (optional) | 1. Add frozen mango chunks to a blender.<br>2. Pour in honey and lemon juice.<br>3. Blend until smooth and creamy.<br>4. Transfer to a container and freeze for 4 hours before serving. |

**Nutritional facts /value (per serving)**

| Cal: 100 | Carbs: 25g | Protein: 1g | Total Fats: 0.6g | Sodium: 1mg |
|---|---|---|---|---|
| Pott: 277mg | Calcium:20mg | Phos: 18mg | Fiber: 3g | Sugar: 20g |

## 9.2  BAKED PEAR WITH CINNAMON AND WALNUTS

| PREPARATION TIME | COOKING TIME | SERVING |
|---|---|---|
| 10 mins | 30 mins | 4 |

| INGREDIENTS | DIRECTIONS |
|---|---|
| 4 pears, halved and cored<br>1 tsp cinnamon<br>¼ cup walnuts, chopped<br>2 tbsp honey (optional) | 1. Set the oven to 355°F (175°C).<br>2. Place pear halves cut-side up in a baking dish.<br>3. Sprinkle with cinnamon and top with chopped walnuts.<br>4. Drizzle with honey, if using.<br>5. Bake for 30 minutes or until pears are tender. |

**Nutritional facts /value (per serving)**

| Cal: 150 | Carbs: 31g | Protein: 2g | Total Fats: 4g | Sodium: 1mg |
|---|---|---|---|---|
| Pott: 210mg | Calcium: 25mg | Phos:30mg | Fiber: 6g | Sugar: 20g |

## 9.3  GRILLED PEACHES WITH GREEK YOGURT

| PREPARATION TIME | COOKING TIME | SERVING |
|---|---|---|
| 10 mins | 10 mins | 4 |

| INGREDIENTS | DIRECTIONS |
|---|---|
| 4 peaches, halved and pitted<br>1 cup Greek yogurt<br>2 tbsp honey (optional)<br>½ tsp cinnamon | 1. Preheat grill to medium-high heat.<br>2. Grill peaches cut-side down for 4-5 minutes.<br>3. Flip and grill for another 4-5 minutes. |

4. Serve with a dollop of Greek yogurt, a drizzle of honey, and a sprinkle of cinnamon.

### Nutritional facts /value (per serving)

| Cal: 100 | Carbs: 19g | Protein: 5g | Total Fats: 1g | Sodium: 15mg |
|---|---|---|---|---|
| Pott: 325mg | Calcium: 60mg | Phos: 45mg | Fiber: 2g | Sugar: 17g |

## 9.4 MANGO COCONUT CHIA PUDDING

| PREPARATION TIME | CHILLING TIME | SERVING |
|---|---|---|
| 15 mins | 3 hrs. | 4 |

**INGREDIENTS**
1 cup coconut milk
¼ cup chia seeds
1 tbsp honey (optional)
1 tsp vanilla extract
2 mangoes, peeled and sliced

**DIRECTIONS**
1. In a bowl, combine coconut milk, chia seeds, honey, and vanilla extract. Stir well to combine.
2. Cover and refrigerate for at least 3 hours or overnight.
3. Serve topped with fresh mango slices.

### Nutritional facts /value (per serving)

| Cal: 220 | Carbs: 30g | Protein: 4g | Total Fats: 10g | Sodium: 15mg |
|---|---|---|---|---|
| Pott: 300mg | Calcium: 150mg | Phos: 100mg | Fiber: 8g | Sugar: 20g |

## 9.5 COCONUT BANANA FREEZE

| PREPARATION TIME | CHILLING TIME | SERVING |
|---|---|---|
| 10 mins | 2hrs. | 6 |

**INGREDIENTS**
3 bananas, sliced and frozen
1 cup coconut milk
1 tsp vanilla extract
Unsweetened shredded coconut for garnish

**DIRECTIONS**
1. Place the frozen banana slices, coconut milk, and vanilla extract in a blender.
2. Blend until smooth and creamy.
3. Serve immediately, garnished with a sprinkle of shredded coconut.

### Nutritional facts /value (per serving)

| Cal: 120 | Carbs: 18g | Protein: 1g | Total Fats: 6g | Sodium: 8mg |
|---|---|---|---|---|
| Pott: 320mg | Calcium: 15mg | Phos: 25mg | Fiber: 3g | Sugar: 10g |

## 9.6  BERRY BLISS PARFAIT

| PREPARATION TIME | COOKING TIME | SERVING |
|---|---|---|
| 15 mins | 0 mins | 4 |

**INGREDIENTS**
2 cups mixed berries (strawberries, blueberries, raspberries)
1 cup Greek yogurt (unsweetened)
2 tbsp honey
½ tsp vanilla extract
¼ cup granola (unsweetened)

**DIRECTIONS**
1. In a bowl, combine the Greek yogurt, honey, and vanilla extract.
2. In serving glasses or bowls, layer the yogurt mixture, berries, and granola.
3. Repeat the layers until all ingredients are used up.
4. Serve immediately, garnished with a sprig of mint if desired.

**Nutritional facts /value (per serving)**

| Cal: 150 | Carbs: 28g | Protein: 5g | Total Fats: 2.5g | Sodium: 30mg |
|---|---|---|---|---|
| Pott: 200mg | Calcium: 100mg | Phos: 85mg | Fiber: 4g | Sugar: 20g |

## 9.7  ALMOND BISCUITS

| PREPARATION TIME | COOKING TIME | SERVING |
|---|---|---|
| 10 mins | 12 mins | 6 |

**INGREDIENTS**
2 cups almond flour
1 egg
¼ cup erythritol or stevia
1 tsp vanilla extract¼ cup granola (unsweetened)

**DIRECTIONS**
1. Preheat your oven to 350°F (180°C).
2. In a bowl, combine all ingredients to form a dough.
3. Form the dough into small round biscuits and place on a lined baking tray.
4. Bake for 12-15 minutes or until golden brown.
5. Allow to cool before serving.

**Nutritional facts /value (per serving)**

| Cal: 140 | Carbs: 5g | Protein: 6g | Total Fats: 12g | Sodium: 11mg |
|---|---|---|---|---|
| Pott: 20mg | Calcium: 60mg | Phos: 96mg | Fiber: 3g | Sugar: 1g |

## 9.8  OAT COOKIES

| PREPARATION TIME | COOKING TIME | SERVING |
|---|---|---|
| 10 mins | 12 mins | 6 |

**INGREDIENTS**
2 cups rolled oats
½ cup unsweetened applesauce
1 tsp cinnamon
1 tbsp chia seeds
2 tbsp honey

**DIRECTIONS**
1. Preheat your oven to 350°F (180°C).
2. In a bowl, mix all ingredients until well combined.

3. Scoop out tbsp-sized portions onto a lined baking tray.
4. Flatten the scoops into cookie shapes and bake for 12-15 minutes or until golden brown.

**Nutritional facts /value (per serving)**

| Cal: 99 | Carbs: 18g | Protein: 3g | Total Fats: 2g | Sodium: 2mg |
|---|---|---|---|---|
| Pott: 96mg | Calcium: 19mg | Phos: 55mg | Fiber: 3g | Sugar: 5g |

## 9.9 COCONUT COOKIES

| PREPARATION TIME | COOKING TIME | SERVING |
|---|---|---|
| 15 mins | 10 mins | 6 |

| INGREDIENTS | DIRECTIONS |
|---|---|
| 2 cups desiccated coconut<br>¼ cup coconut oil, melted<br>¼ cup honey<br>1 egg<br>1 tsp vanilla extract | 1. Preheat your oven to 350°F (180°C).<br>2. In a bowl, combine all ingredients to form a cohesive mixture.<br>3. Using a tbsp, scoop portions onto a lined baking tray, forming cookie shapes.<br>4. Bake for 10-12 minutes or until edges are golden brown. |

**Nutritional facts /value (per serving)**

| Cal: 205 | Carbs: 10g | Protein: 2g | Total Fats: 18g | Sodium: 9mg |
|---|---|---|---|---|
| Pott: 68mg | Calcium: 8mg | Phos: 32mg | Fiber: 5g | Sugar: 5g |

## 9.10 LEMON POPPY SEED COOKIES

| PREPARATION TIME | COOKING TIME | SERVING |
|---|---|---|
| 15 mins | 12 mins | 6 |

| INGREDIENTS | DIRECTIONS |
|---|---|
| 1 and ½ cups almond flour<br>Zest of 1 lemon<br>2 tbsp lemon juice<br>¼ cup coconut oil, melted<br>¼ cup honey<br>1 tbsp poppy seeds<br>½ tsp baking soda | 1. Preheat your oven to 350°F (180°C).<br>2. In a bowl, combine all ingredients to form a cohesive mixture.<br>3. Using a tbsp, scoop portions onto a lined baking tray, forming cookie shapes.<br>4. Bake for 10-12 minutes or until edges are golden brown. |

**Nutritional facts /value (per serving)**

| Cal: 200 | Carbs: 11g | Protein: 5g | Total Fats: 17g | Sodium: 85mg |
|---|---|---|---|---|
| Pott: 60mg | Calcium: 55mg | Phos: 90mg | Fiber: 3g | Sugar: 8g |

## 9.11   COCONUT FLAXSEED COOKIES

| PREPARATION TIME | COOKING TIME | SERVING |
|---|---|---|
| 15 mins | 12 mins | 6 |

### INGREDIENTS

1 cup coconut flour
½ cup ground flaxseed
¼ cup melted coconut oil
¼ cup maple syrup or sugar-free syrup
1 tsp vanilla extract
½ tsp baking soda
2 eggs
A pinch of salt

### DIRECTIONS

1. Begin by preheating your oven to 350°F (180°C).
2. In one bowl, blend together coconut flour, ground flaxseed, and baking soda.
3. In a separate bowl, whisk together coconut oil, maple syrup, vanilla extract, and eggs.
4. Merge the wet and dry ingredients, thoroughly mixing to create a cookie dough.
5. Scoop out tbsp-sized portions onto a lined baking tray, gently flattening each with a fork.
6. Bake for 10-12 minutes or until edges are golden.

**Nutritional facts /value (per serving)**

| Cal: 190 | Carbs: 14g | Protein: 5g | Total Fats: 15g | Sodium: 100mg |
|---|---|---|---|---|
| Pott: 90mg | Calcium: 45mg | Phos: 70mg | Fiber: 6g | Sugar: 9g |

## 9.12   WALNUT & CINNAMON BISCUITS

| PREPARATION TIME | COOKING TIME | SERVING |
|---|---|---|
| 15 mins | 15 mins | 6 |

### INGREDIENTS

1 and ½ cups walnut meal
½ tsp ground cinnamon
¼ cup melted butter
¼ cup erythritol or another sugar substitute
1 egg
½ tsp baking soda
A pinch of salt

### DIRECTIONS

1. Preheat the oven to 350°F (180°C).
2. In a bowl, mix walnut meal, cinnamon, baking soda, and salt.
3. Stir in the melted butter, erythritol, and egg until well combined.
4. Drop tbsp of the mixture onto a lined baking tray, shaping them into biscuits.
5. Bake for 12-15 minutes or until slightly golden around the edges.

**Nutritional facts /value (per serving)**

| Cal: 205 | Carbs: 4g | Protein: 5g | Total Fats: 20g | Sodium: 105mg |
|---|---|---|---|---|
| Pott: 85mg | Calcium: 4mg | Phos: 75mg | Fiber: 2g | Sugar: 1g |

## 9.13   LEMON AND CHIA SEED MUFFINS

| PREPARATION TIME | COOKING TIME | SERVING |
|---|---|---|
| 15 mins | 20 mins | 6 |

### INGREDIENTS

2 cups almond flour
½ cup erythritol or stevia
1 tsp baking powder
Zest and juice of 1 lemon
4 eggs
4 tbsp melted unsalted butter
2 tbsp chia seeds

### DIRECTIONS

1. Preheat the oven to 350°F (180°C).
2. In a bowl, combine the almond flour, erythritol, and baking powder.
3. Add in the lemon zest, lemon juice, eggs, and melted butter. Mix until well combined.
4. Stir in the chia seeds.
5. Divide the mixture into a greased muffin tray.
6. Bake for 20-25 minutes or until golden and a toothpick comes out clean.

### Nutritional facts /value (per serving)

| Cal: 200 | Carbs: 7g | Protein: 8g | Total Fats: 17g | Sodium: 100mg |
|---|---|---|---|---|
| Pott: 60mg | Calcium: 100mg | Phos: 80mg | Fiber: 4g | Sugar: 1g |

## 9.14   LIGHT APPLE CINNAMON CAKE

| PREPARATION TIME | COOKING TIME | SERVING |
|---|---|---|
| 20 mins | 30 mins | 8 |

### INGREDIENTS

2 cups oat flour
½ cup unsweetened applesauce
¼ cup erythritol or stevia
1 tsp baking powder
½ tsp ground cinnamon
2 apples, peeled and diced
2 eggs
4 tbsp melted unsalted butter

### DIRECTIONS

1. Preheat the oven to 350°F (180°C).
2. In a bowl, mix the oat flour, erythritol, baking powder, and cinnamon.
3. Stir in the applesauce, eggs, and melted butter until combined.
4. Fold in the diced apples.
5. Transfer the mixture to a greased and lined cake tin.
6. Bake for 30-35 minutes or until a toothpick comes out clean.

### Nutritional facts /value (per serving)

| Cal: 190 | Carbs: 27g | Protein: 5g | Total Fats: 7g | Sodium: 90mg |
|---|---|---|---|---|
| Pott: 115mg | Calcium: 60mg | Phos: 85mg | Fiber: 4g | Sugar: 9g |

## 9.15   BANANA WALNUT MINI CAKES

| PREPARATION TIME | COOKING TIME | SERVING |
|---|---|---|
| 15 mins | 25 mins | 6 |

### INGREDIENTS

3 ripe bananas, mashed
1 ½ cups almond flour
½ cup walnuts, chopped
¼ cup coconut oil, melted
¼ cup erythritol or stevia
1 tsp vanilla extract
1 tsp baking powder
½ tsp cinnamon

### DIRECTIONS

1. Preheat the oven to 350°F (180°C).
2. In a bowl, combine the mashed bananas, almond flour, erythritol, baking powder, and cinnamon.
3. Mix in the melted coconut oil and vanilla extract.
4. Stir in the chopped walnuts.
5. Transfer the mixture into mini cake molds or a greased muffin tray.
6. Bake for 25-30 minutes or until a toothpick comes out clean.

**Nutritional facts /value (per serving)**

| Cal: 210 | Carbs: 15g | Protein: 6g | Total Fats: 15 | Sodium: 80mg |
|---|---|---|---|---|
| Pott: 210mg | Calcium: 60 | Phos: 90mg | Fiber: 4g | Sugar: 7g |

## 9.16   PUMPKIN SPICE MINI CAKES

| PREPARATION TIME | COOKING TIME | SERVING |
|---|---|---|
| 20 mins | 30 mins | 6 |

### INGREDIENTS

1 ½ cups pumpkin puree
2 cups almond flour
½ cup erythritol or stevia
2 tsp pumpkin pie spice
1 tsp baking soda
2 eggs
¼ cup unsweetened almond milk
¼ cup coconut oil, melted

### DIRECTIONS

1. Start by preheating your oven to 350°F (180°C).
2. In one bowl, combine almond flour, erythritol, pumpkin pie spice, and baking soda.
3. In another bowl, blend together the pumpkin puree, eggs, almond milk, and melted coconut oil.
4. Combine the wet ingredients with the dry ingredients, mixing until a cohesive batter forms.
5. Transfer the batter into greased mini cake molds or use a muffin tray.
6. Bake for approximately 30-35 minutes, or until a toothpick inserted into the center emerges clean.
7. Allow the cakes to cool slightly before serving.

**Nutritional facts /value (per serving)**

| Cal: 200 | Carbs: 15g | Protein: 8g | Total Fats: 14g | Sodium: 120mg |
|---|---|---|---|---|
| Pott: 180mg | Calcium: 99mg | Phos: 100mg | Fiber: 6g | Sugar: 3g |

## 9.17 BLUEBERRY OAT MUFFINS

| PREPARATION TIME | COOKING TIME | SERVING |
|---|---|---|
| 20 mins | 25 mins | 6 |

### INGREDIENTS

1 cup whole wheat flour
1 cup rolled oats
½ cup almond flour
2 tsp baking powder
½ tsp baking soda
¼ tsp salt
¼ cup honey or pure maple syrup
2 tbsp coconut oil, melted
1 cup unsweetened almond milk
1 tsp vanilla extract
1 large egg or flaxseed egg (1 tbsp flaxseed mixed with 2.5 tbsp water)
1 cup fresh blueberries

### DIRECTIONS

1. Preheat the oven to 350°F (175°C). Grease or line a muffin tin with paper liners.
2. In a large mixing bowl, whisk together the whole wheat flour, rolled oats, almond flour, baking powder, baking soda, and salt.
3. In another bowl, mix the honey or maple syrup, melted coconut oil, almond milk, vanilla extract, and egg until well combined.
4. Pour the wet ingredients into the dry and mix just until combined. Do not overmix.
5. Gently fold in the blueberries.
6. Evenly divide the batter among the muffin cups.
7. Bake for 22-25 minutes or until a toothpick inserted into the center comes out clean.
8. Let the muffins cool in the pan for 5 minutes, then transfer them to a wire rack to cool completely.

### Nutritional facts /value (per serving)

| | | | | |
|---|---|---|---|---|
| **Cal:** 210 | **Carbs:** 28g | **Protein:** 5g | **Total Fats:** 8g | **Sodium:** 220mg |
| **Pott:** 185mg | **Calcium:** 100mg | **Phos:** 77mg | **Fiber:** 4g | **Sugar:** 10g |

## 9.18 MATCHA & ALMOND CAKE

| PREPARATION TIME | COOKING TIME | SERVING |
|---|---|---|
| 20 mins | 30 mins | 6 |

### INGREDIENTS

1 ½ cups almond flour
2 tbsp matcha green tea powder
1 tsp baking powder
¼ tsp salt
3 large eggs, room temperature
1/3 cup coconut milk (fat free)
¼ cup melted coconut oil
¼ cup honey or maple syrup

### DIRECTIONS

1. Preheat the oven to 350°F (175°C) and grease an 8-inch cake pan.
2. In a mixing bowl, whisk together the almond flour, matcha powder, baking powder, and salt.
3. In another bowl, beat the eggs and then add the coconut milk, melted coconut oil,

1 tsp almond extract

honey or maple syrup, and almond extract. Mix well.

4. Gently fold the dry ingredients into the wet mixture until well combined.
5. Pour the batter into the prepared cake pan and spread it evenly.
6. Bake for 25-30 minutes or until the cake is firm to the touch and a toothpick inserted into the center comes out clean.
7. Remove from the oven and let it cool in the pan for about 10 minutes, then transfer to a wire rack to cool completely before serving.

**Nutritional facts /value (per serving)**

| **Cal:** 210 | **Carbs:** 14g | **Protein:** 6g | **Total Fats:** 15g | **Sodium:** 120mg |
|---|---|---|---|---|
| **Pott:** 70mg | **Calcium:** 80g | **Phos:** 85mg | **Fiber:** 4g | **Sugar:** 11g |

## 9.19   BANANA & AVOCADO ICE CREAM

| PREPARATION TIME | FREEZING TIME | SERVING |
|---|---|---|
| 10 mins | 3 hrs. | 4 |

**INGREDIENTS**

3 ripe bananas, peeled and sliced
1 ripe avocado, peeled and pitted
2 tbsp almond butter (or any nut butter of choice)
1 tsp pure vanilla extract
A pinch of salt
1 tbsp chia seeds (optional for added fiber and texture)
2 tbsp maple syrup or honey (optional for added sweetness)

**DIRECTIONS**

1. Place the banana slices in a plastic bag and freeze for at least 2 hours.
2. In a blender or food processor, combine the frozen bananas, avocado, almond butter, vanilla extract, salt, and sweetener (if using). Blend until smooth and creamy.
3. If you desire a firmer texture, fold in chia seeds, and transfer the mixture to a container and freeze for another hour.
4. Serve immediately for a soft-serve consistency or freeze for an additional 1-2 hours for a firmer texture. Scoop into bowls and enjoy!

**Nutritional facts /value (per serving)**

| **Cal:** 220 | **Carbs:** 28g | **Protein:** 3g | **Total Fats:** 12g | **Sodium:** 10mg |
|---|---|---|---|---|
| **Pott:** 600mg | **Calcium:** 40g | **Phos:** 80mg | **Fiber:** 7g | **Sugar:** 14g |

## 9.20    BERRY BLISS ICE CREAM

| PREPARATION TIME | FREEZING TIME | SERVING |
|---|---|---|
| 10 mins | 3 hrs. | 6 |

### INGREDIENTS

4 cups mixed berries (strawberries, blueberries, raspberries), frozen
1 can (400ml) coconut milk, fat free
2 tbsp fresh lemon juice
2 tbsp flaxseeds, ground
1 tsp vanilla extract
2 tbsp honey or maple syrup (optional)

### DIRECTIONS

1. In a blender or food processor, add the frozen mixed berries, coconut milk, and lemon juice.
2. Blend on high until smooth and creamy, adding more coconut milk if necessary.
3. Stir in the ground flaxseeds and vanilla extract. If using, add in the honey or maple syrup and blend until well combined.
4. Transfer the mixture into an airtight container and freeze for about 3 hours, or until firm.
5. Before serving, let it sit at room temperature for a few minutes to soften. Scoop into bowls and enjoy your homemade dairy-free ice cream.

### Nutritional facts /value (per serving)

| Cal: 200 | Carbs: 18g | Protein: 2g | Total Fats: 15g | Sodium: 15mg |
|---|---|---|---|---|
| Pott: 210mg | Calcium: 25g | Phos: 45mg | Fiber: 5g | Sugar: 10g |

## 9.21    MINT & SPINACH ICE CREAM

| PREPARATION TIME | FREEZING TIME | SERVING |
|---|---|---|
| 10 mins | 4 hrs. | 4 |

### INGREDIENTS

1 ripe avocado, peeled and pitted
1 cup fresh spinach leaves
1 can (400ml) coconut milk, fat free
½ cup fresh mint leaves
¼ cup honey or maple syrup (optional)
2 tsp vanilla extract
1 tbsp lime juice

### DIRECTIONS

1. In a blender, add the avocado, coconut milk, spinach, mint leaves, honey (if using), vanilla extract, and lime juice.
2. Blend until the mixture is smooth and creamy.
3. Pour the mixture into an airtight container and freeze for at least 4 hours, or until solid.
4. Allow to soften for a few minutes at room temperature before scooping into bowls to serve.

### Nutritional facts /value (per serving)

| Cal: 230 | Carbs: 18g | Protein: 3g | Total Fats: 18g | Sodium: 20mg |
|---|---|---|---|---|
| Pott: 550mg | Calcium: 45g | Phos: 65mg | Fiber: 6g | Sugar: 10g |

## 9.22   CHOCOLATE & ALMOND BUTTER ICE CREAM

| PREPARATION TIME | FREEZING TIME | SERVING |
|---|---|---|
| 10 mins | 4 hrs. | 6 |

### INGREDIENTS
3 bananas, sliced and frozen
¼ cup cocoa powder, unsweetened
½ cup almond butter
1 can (400ml) coconut milk, fat free
2 tbsp honey or maple syrup (optional)
1 tsp almond extract

### DIRECTIONS
1. Place the frozen banana slices, cocoa powder, almond butter, and coconut milk in a food processor or blender.
2. Blend until smooth and creamy, adding more coconut milk if necessary.
3. Add the honey (if using) and almond extract and blend until well incorporated.
4. Transfer the mixture to an airtight container and freeze for at least 4 hours, or until solid

**Nutritional facts /value (per serving)**

| Cal: 280 | Carbs: 24g | Protein: 7g | Total Fats: 20g | Sodium: 10mg |
|---|---|---|---|---|
| Pott: 540mg | Calcium: 80g | Phos: 100mg | Fiber: 6g | Sugar: 14g |

## 9.23   GINGER & TURMERIC SPICE ICE CREAM

| PREPARATION TIME | FREEZING TIME | SERVING |
|---|---|---|
| 10 mins | 4 hrs. | 4 |

### INGREDIENTS
2 ripe bananas, sliced and frozen
1 inch fresh ginger, peeled and grated
1 tsp ground turmeric
1 can (400ml) coconut milk, fat free
2 tbsp honey or maple syrup (optional)
1 tsp vanilla extract
A pinch of ground cinnamon

### DIRECTIONS
1. Place the frozen banana slices in a blender or food processor.
2. Add the grated ginger, ground turmeric, coconut milk, and vanilla extract to the blender.
3. Blend until the mixture becomes creamy and smooth.
4. Add honey (if using) and a pinch of cinnamon, and blend until all ingredients are well incorporated.
5. Transfer the mixture to an airtight container and freeze for at least 4 hours, until solid.
6. Allow the ice cream to soften at room temperature for a few minutes before serving.

**Nutritional facts /value (per serving)**

| Cal: 200 | Carbs: 24g | Protein: 2g | Total Fats: 13g | Sodium: 10mg |
|---|---|---|---|---|
| Pott: 370mg | Calcium: 40g | Phos: 55mg | Fiber: 3g | Sugar: 16g |

## 9.24 SPICED BUTTERNUT SQUASH ICE CREAM

| PREPARATION TIME | FREEZING TIME | SERVING |
|---|---|---|
| 20 mins | 4-6 hrs. | 4 |

### INGREDIENTS
2 cups butternut squash, roasted and mashed
1 can (400ml) coconut milk
¼ cup maple syrup
½ tsp nutmeg powder
1 tbsp vanilla extract
1 tsp cinnamon powder

### DIRECTIONS
1. Blend the roasted butternut squash until smooth.
2. Add coconut milk, maple syrup, cinnamon, nutmeg, and vanilla extract to the blender and blend until well combined.
3. Pour the mixture into an ice cream maker and churn according to manufacturer's instructions.
4. Transfer the ice cream to an airtight container and freeze for at least 4-6 hours before serving.

### Nutritional facts /value (per serving)

| Cal: 220 | Carbs: 25g | Protein: 2g | Total Fats: 14g | Sodium: 20mg |
|---|---|---|---|---|
| Pott: 400mg | Calcium: 40g | Phos: 55mg | Fiber: 3g | Sugar: 15g |

# 10.  SPECIAL DIETARY NEEDS

## 10.1  BAKED SALMON WITH QUINOA AND DILL

| PREPARATION TIME | COOKING TIME | SERVING |
|---|---|---|
| 10 mins | 20 mins | 4 |

| INGREDIENTS | DIRECTIONS |
|---|---|
| 4 salmon fillets<br>1 cup quinoa, rinsed and drained<br>2 cups low-sodium chicken or vegetable broth<br>1 lemon, zest and juice<br>2 tbsp fresh dill, chopped<br>Salt to taste<br>Black pepper to taste<br>Olive oil for drizzling | 1. Set the temperature of the oven to 375°F (190°C).<br>2. Marinate salmon fillets with salt, pepper, and lemon zest.<br>3. Bake the salmon for about 15-20 minutes or until cooked through and flaky.<br>4. Meanwhile, add quinoa and chicken or vegetable broth in a pot. Bring to a boil, cover, and simmer for about 15 minutes on low heat.<br>5. Add lemon juice and chopped fresh dill.<br>6. Ready to serve |

**Nutritional facts /value (per serving)**

| Cal: 350 | Carbs: 45g | Protein: 30g | Total Fats: 10g | Sodium: 150mg |
|---|---|---|---|---|
| Pott: 650mg | Calcium: 40mg | Phos: 360mg | Fiber: 3g | Sugar: 2g |

## 10.2  GRILLED CHICKEN WITH CAULIFLOWER

| PREPARATION TIME | COOKING TIME | SERVING |
|---|---|---|
| 15 mins | 20 mins | 4 |

| INGREDIENTS | DIRECTIONS |
|---|---|
| 1 head cauliflower, cut into florets<br>2 cloves garlic, minced<br>Two tbsp of olive oil<br>Salt<br>4 boneless, skinless chicken breasts<br>1 tsp paprika<br>1 tsp dried thyme<br>Black pepper<br>Cooked brown rice or quinoa, for serving | 1. Steam or boil cauliflower, add to the food processor.<br>2. Add minced garlic, salt, pepper, and oil in the cauliflower and mash until smooth.<br>3. Pre heat a grill or grill pan on medium heat.<br>4. Marinate chicken with paprika, thyme, salt and pepper.<br>5. Grill the chicken for about 6-8 minutes per side and serve with mashed cauliflower. |

**Nutritional facts /value (per serving)**

| Cal: 330 | Carbs: 15g | Protein: 40g | Total Fats: 12g | Sodium: 380mg |
|---|---|---|---|---|
| Pott: 1050mg | Calcium: 150mg | Phos: 350mg | Fiber: 5g | Sugar: 5g |

## 10.3 TURKEY BOLOGNESE AND SPAGHETTI SQUASH

| PREPARATION TIME | COOKING TIME | SERVING |
|---|---|---|
| 15 mins | 45 mins | 4 |

| INGREDIENTS | DIRECTIONS |
|---|---|
| 1 spaghetti squash<br>1 lb. lean ground turkey<br>1 onion, chopped<br>2 cloves garlic, minced<br>1 can (15 oz) tomatoes, crushed<br>1 tsp basil, dried<br>1 tsp oregano, dried<br>Salt to taste<br>Black pepper to taste<br>Olive oil for sautéing | 1. Preheat the oven to 375°F (190°C).<br>2. Cut the spaghetti squash lengthwise and remove the seeds.<br>3. Roast for about 30-40 minutes.<br>4. Meanwhile, heat olive oil over medium heat. Add chopped onion and sauté until translucent.<br>5. Add minced garlic and turkey. Cook until the turkey is browned and cooked through, breaking it into crumbles<br>6. Add crushed tomatoes, dried basil, dried oregano, salt, and pepper to the pan. Cook for about 15 minutes.<br>7. Once the squash is d1, scrape the flesh with a fork to create spaghetti-like strands.<br>8. Serve the turkey Bolognese over the spaghetti squash |

| Nutritional facts /value (per serving) | | | | |
|---|---|---|---|---|
| **Cal:** 320 | **Carbs:** 30g | **Protein:** 25g | **Total Fats:** 10g | **Sodium:** 520mg |
| **Pott:** 850mg | **Calcium:** 60mg | **Phos:** 290mg | **Fiber:** 8g | **Sugar:** 6g |

## 10.4 MASALA OATS WITH MIXED GREENS

| PREPARATION TIME | COOKING TIME | SERVING |
|---|---|---|
| 15 mins | 20 mins | 4 |

| INGREDIENTS | DIRECTIONS |
|---|---|
| 2 tbsp olive oil<br>1 cup oats, rinsed and drained<br>2 cups vegetable broth<br>2 cups mixed vegetables (bell peppers, broccoli, spinach, carrots, etc.), chopped<br>Salt to taste<br>2 cloves garlic, minced<br>2 tbsp gluten-free soy sauce or tamari<br>Pepper to taste | 1. Boil oats in vegetable broth for 15 minutes.<br>2. Meanwhile, heat olive oil in a large wok. Add minced garlic and chopped mixed vegetables. Stir-fry for about 5-7 minutes.<br>3. Add gluten-free soy sauce, salt, and pepper. Cook for another 2 minutes.<br>4. Fluff the cooked quinoa with a fork and add it to the wok with the stir-fried vegetables. Toss to combine.<br>5. Serve the quinoa and vegetable stir-fry hot. |

**Nutritional facts /value (per serving)**

| Cal: 240 | Carbs: 45g | Protein: 8g | Total Fats: 15g | Sodium: 500mg |
|---|---|---|---|---|
| Pott: 480mg | Calcium: 60mg | Phos: 160mg | Fiber: 6g | Sugar: 6g |

## 10.5 GRILLED SHRIMPS WITH QUINOA SALAD

| PREPARATION TIME | COOKING TIME | SERVING |
|---|---|---|
| 10 mins | 20 mins | 4 |

| INGREDIENTS | DIRECTIONS |
|---|---|
| 1 lb. large shrimp, peeled and deveined<br>Zest and juice of 1 lemon<br>2 tbsp fresh parsley, chopped<br>2 tbsp fresh basil, chopped<br>2 cloves garlic, minced<br>Olive oil for grilling<br>1 cup quinoa, rinsed and drained<br>2 cups low-sodium vegetable broth<br>1 cucumber, diced<br>1 cup cherry tomatoes, halved<br>¼ cup red onion, finely chopped<br>2 tbsp fresh mint, chopped<br>2 tbsp fresh dill, chopped<br>2 tbsp olive oil<br>Salt and black pepper to taste | 1. In a bowl, combine lemon zest, lemon juice, chopped fresh parsley, chopped fresh basil, minced garlic, salt, and pepper and marinate shrimps in it for 10 minutes.<br>2. Preheat a grill or grill pan over medium-high heat. Thread the shrimp onto skewers<br>3. Rill the shrimps for 2-3 minutes each side.<br>4. For quinoa salad boil quinoa with vegetable broth for 15 minutes<br>5. Add boiled quinoa diced cucumber, halved cherry tomatoes, finely chopped red onion, mint, chopped dill, olive oil, salt and pepper.<br>6. Serve quinoa salad with shrimps. |

**Nutritional facts /value (per serving)**

| Cal: 250 | Carbs: 30g | Protein: 18g | Total Fats: 7g | Sodium: 380mg |
|---|---|---|---|---|
| Pott: 540mg | Calcium: 60mg | Phos: 180mg | Fiber: 4g | Sugar: 2g |

## 10.6 BLACK BEAN BOWL WITH SWEET POTATO

| PREPARATION TIME | COOKING TIME | SERVING |
|---|---|---|
| 15 mins | 20 mins | 2 |

| INGREDIENTS | DIRECTIONS |
|---|---|
| 1 cup quinoa, rinsed<br>2 cups vegetable broth<br>2 medium sweet potatoes diced<br>1 can (15 oz) black beans, drained and rinsed<br>1 cup corn kernels<br>½ red onion, finely chopped<br>2 tbsp fresh cilantro, chopped<br>1 tsp cumin<br>1 tsp chili powder<br>Olive oil for roasting | 1. Preheat the oven to 400°F (200°C).<br>2. Mix diced sweet potatoes with olive oil, cumin, chili powder, salt, and pepper. Put them out on a baking sheet and roast for about 15-20 minutes<br>3. Meanwhile, add quinoa and vegetable broth in a pot and boil for 15 minutes<br>4. Fluff the cooked quinoa with a fork.<br>5. In a large bowl, mix the cooked quinoa, roasted sweet potatoes, black beans, corn kernels, finely chopped red onion, and fresh cilantro. |

6. Serve the sweet potato and black bean quinoa bowl.

**Nutritional facts /value (per serving)**

| Cal: 390 | Carbs: 77g | Protein: 15g | Total Fats: 4g | Sodium: 480mg |
|---|---|---|---|---|
| Pott: 900mg | Calcium: 80mg | Phos: 280mg | Fiber: 13g | Sugar: 7g |

## 10.7 MEDITERRANEAN CHICKPEA SALAD

| PREPARATION TIME | COOKING TIME | SERVING |
|---|---|---|
| 15 mins | 0 mins | 2 |

| INGREDIENTS | DIRECTIONS |
|---|---|
| 2 cups chickpeas, canned<br>1 cup cucumber, diced<br>1 cup cherry tomatoes, halved<br>¼ cup red onion, chopped<br>¼ cup fresh parsley, chopped<br>¼ cup Kalamata olives, pitted and sliced<br>2 tbsp extra-virgin olive oil<br>2 tbsp lemon juice<br>1 tsp dried oregano | 1. Mix chickpeas, diced cucumber, halved cherry tomatoes, finely chopped red onion, chopped fresh parsley, and sliced Kalamata olives in a bowl.<br>2. In a separate bowl, whisk together extra-virgin olive oil, lemon juice, dried oregano, salt, and pepper.<br>3. Drizzle the dressing over the salad and toss to coat.<br>4. Serve the Mediterranean chickpea salad cold. |

**Nutritional facts /value (per serving)**

| Cal: 380 | Carbs: 45g | Protein: 13g | Total Fats: 18g | Sodium: 650mg |
|---|---|---|---|---|
| Pott: 760mg | Calcium: 90mg | Phos: 200mg | Fiber: 12g | Sugar: 6g |

## 10.8 STUFFED PORTOBELLO MUSHROOMS

| PREPARATION TIME | COOKING TIME | SERVING |
|---|---|---|
| 15 mins | 20 mins | 2 |

| INGREDIENTS | DIRECTIONS |
|---|---|
| 4 large Portobello mushrooms<br>2 cups fresh spinach, chopped<br>1 cup cremini mushrooms, finely chopped<br>½ cup onion, chopped<br>2 cloves garlic, minced<br>¼ cup nutritional yeast (for a cheesy flavor)<br>2 tbsp olive oil<br><br>Fresh basil, for garnish | 1. Preheat the oven to 375°F (190°C).<br>2. Remove the stems from the Portobello mushrooms and scrape out the gills. Brush the mushroom caps lightly with olive oil.<br>3. In a pan, heat 1 tbsp of olive oil over medium heat. Add finely chopped cremini mushrooms, minced garlic, and finely chopped onion. Cook until the mushrooms release their moisture and the onion is translucent.<br>4. Add chopped fresh spinach and continue to cook until it wilts.<br>5. Remove the pan from heat and add nutritional yeast. Season with . |

6. Stuff each Portobello mushroom cap with the spinach and mushroom mixture.
7. Bake in the preheated oven for about 15-20 minutes, or until the mushrooms are tender.
8. Garnish with fresh basil leaves before serving.

**Nutritional facts /value (per serving)**

| Cal: 180 | Carbs: 20g | Protein: 12g | Total Fats: 18g | Sodium: 60mg |
|---|---|---|---|---|
| Pott: 1120mg | Calcium: 50mg | Phos: 290mg | Fiber: 7g | Sugar: 5g |

## 10.9 EGGPLANT AND LENTIL CURRY

| PREPARATION TIME | COOKING TIME | SERVING |
|---|---|---|
| 10 mins | 0 mins | 1 |

### INGREDIENTS

1 large eggplant, diced
1 cup brown lentils
2 cups low-sodium vegetable broth
1 can (14 oz) tomatoes, diced
1 onion, chopped
2 cloves garlic, minced
1 tsp curry powder
1 tsp ground turmeric
1 tsp ground cumin
½ tsp ground coriander
¼ tsp cayenne pepper (adjust to taste)
2 tbsp olive oil

### DIRECTIONS

1. Sauté onions in olive oil over medium heat until translucent.
2. Add minced garlic, curry powder, ground turmeric, ground cumin, ground coriander, and cayenne pepper. Cook for a minute until fragrant.
3. Add diced eggplant and sauté for about 5-7 minutes until it begins to soften.
4. Add lentils, low-sodium vegetable broth, and diced tomatoes. Bring to a boil, then reduce heat, cover, and simmer for about 20-25 minutes, or until the lentils are tender.
5. Taste and adjust the seasoning with salt and pepper if needed.

**Nutritional facts /value (per serving)**

| Cal: 330 | Carbs: 58g | Protein: 16g | Total Fats: 6g | Sodium: 650mg |
|---|---|---|---|---|
| Pott: 1120mg | Calcium: 60mg | Phos: 310mg | Fiber: 20g | Sugar: 13g |

## 10.10 VEGAN CHICKPEA AND SPINACH

| PREPARATION TIME | COOKING TIME | SERVING |
|---|---|---|
| 15 mins | 20 mins | 2 |

## INGREDIENTS

1 cup canned chickpeas, drained and rinsed
2 cups spinach
2 cloves garlic, minced
2 tbsp low-sodium soy sauce
2 tbsp sesame oil
1 tsp ginger, grated
Olive oil for sautéing

## DIRECTIONS

1. Heat olive oil in a large wok over medium-flame. Add minced garlic and grated ginger. Sauté for about 30 seconds until fragrant.
2. Add spinach and stir-fry for about 5-7 minutes.
3. Add canned chickpeas and continue to cook for another 2 minutes.
4. In a small bowl, mix low-sodium soy sauce or tamari with sesame oil.
5. Pour the sauce over the stir-fry, toss to coat, and cook for another 2 minutes to combine flavors.
6. Season with .

### Nutritional facts /value (per serving)

| Cal: 290 | Carbs: 34g | Protein: 11g | Total Fats: 14g | Sodium: 750mg |
|---|---|---|---|---|
| Pott: 470mg | Calcium: 60mg | Phos: 160mg | Fiber: 7g | Sugar: 8g |

## 10.11 LOW CARB GRILLED CHICKEN SALAD

| PREPARATION TIME | COOKING TIME | SERVING |
|---|---|---|
| 20 mins | 15 mins | 4 |

## INGREDIENTS

4 boneless, skinless chicken breasts
1 lemon, zested and juiced
2 garlic cloves, minced
2 tsp dried oregano
Mixed salad greens
1 cucumber, sliced
1 cup cherry tomatoes, halved

## DIRECTIONS

1. Marinate the chicken breasts with lemon zest, lemon juice, garlic, and oregano. Let it marinate for at least 15 minutes.
2. Preheat the grill and cook the chicken for about 6-7 minutes on each side or until fully cooked.
3. In a large bowl, combine salad greens, cucumber, and cherry tomatoes.
4. Slice the grilled chicken and place it on top of the salad.

### Nutritional facts /value (per serving)

| Cal: 220 | Carbs: 8g | Protein: 30g | Total Fats: 6g | Sodium: 80mg |
|---|---|---|---|---|
| Pott: 600mg | Calcium: 50mg | Phos: 250mg | Fiber: 3g | Sugar: 4g |

## *10.12 KETO-FRIENDLY BAKED SALMON*

| PREPARATION TIME | COOKING TIME | SERVING |
|---|---|---|
| 15 mins | 20 mins | 4 |

| INGREDIENTS | DIRECTIONS |
|---|---|
| 4 salmon fillets<br>2 tbsp fresh dill, chopped<br>2 tbsp fresh parsley, chopped<br>1 lemon, sliced<br>1 tbsp olive oil | 1. Preheat your oven to 400°F (200°C).<br>2. Place the salmon fillets on a baking sheet lined with parchment paper.<br>3. In a bowl, mix the dill, parsley, olive oil, salt, and pepper. Spread this mixture on top of the salmon fillets.<br>4. Top with lemon slices and bake for about 15-20 minutes or until the salmon is cooked through.<br>5. Serve with a side of steamed vegetables or a green salad. |

**Nutritional facts /value (per serving)**

| Cal: 300 | Carbs: 1g | Protein: 35g | Total Fats: 7g | Sodium: 60mg |
|---|---|---|---|---|
| Pott: 810mg | Calcium: 30mg | Phos: 390mg | Fiber: 0g | Sugar: 0g |

## *10.13 LOW CARB STEAMED FISH WITH SCALLIONS*

| PREPARATION TIME | COOKING TIME | SERVING |
|---|---|---|
| 15 mins | 20 mins | 4 |

| INGREDIENTS | DIRECTIONS |
|---|---|
| 4 cups mixed vegetables (like broccoli, cauliflower, and carrots)<br>1 tbsp olive oil<br>1 tsp dried herbs (like rosemary or thyme)<br>2 tbsp balsamic vinegar | 1. Preheat the oven to 400°F (200°C).<br>2. Toss the mixed vegetables with olive oil, herbs, salt, and pepper.<br>3. Spread the vegetables on a baking tray in a single layer.<br>4. Roast for about 20 minutes or until the vegetables are tender and slightly caramelized.<br>5. Drizzle the roasted vegetables with balsamic vinegar before serving. |

**Nutritional facts /value (per serving)**

| Cal: 90 | Carbs: 14g | Protein: 3g | Total Fats: 3g | Sodium: 55mg |
|---|---|---|---|---|
| Pott: 650mg | Calcium: 20mg | Phos: 440mg | Fiber: 5g | Sugar: 7g |

## 10.14 KETO-FRIENDLY CAULIFLOWER FRIED RICE

| PREPARATION TIME | COOKING TIME | SERVING |
|---|---|---|
| 15 mins | 10 mins | 4 |

### INGREDIENTS

1 medium cauliflower head, riced (about 4 cups)
1 cup mixed vegetables (peas, carrots, corn), fresh or frozen
2 green onions, chopped
2 garlic cloves, minced
½-inch fresh ginger, minced
2 large eggs, beaten
2 tbsp low-sodium soy sauce
1 tbsp olive oil
1 tsp sesame oil
Fresh cilantro or parsley for garnish (optional)

### DIRECTIONS

1. Wash the cauliflower and cut it into florets. Using a food processor or a grater, rice the cauliflower until it resembles small grains.
2. Heat olive oil in a large skillet or wok over medium heat.
3. Add the minced garlic and ginger, and sauté for about 1 minute or until fragrant.
4. Add the mixed vegetables and cook for 5-7 minutes, until they are softened but still vibrant.
5. Push the vegetables to one side of the skillet and pour the beaten eggs on the other side. Scramble the eggs with a spatula, then mix them with the vegetables.
6. Stir in the cauliflower rice and mix well.
7. Pour the soy sauce and sesame oil over the mixture, and stir to combine.
8. Cook for another 3-5 minutes, until the cauliflower is tender but not mushy.
9. Garnish with chopped green onions and fresh cilantro or parsley before serving.

**Nutritional facts /value (per serving)**

| Cal: 150 | Carbs: 14g | Protein: 6g | Total Fats: 8g | Sodium: 300mg |
|---|---|---|---|---|
| Pott: 500mg | Calcium: 50mg | Phos: 100mg | Fiber: 4g | Sugar: 4g |

## 10.15 LOW CARB STUFFED CABBAGE ROLLS

| PREPARATION TIME | COOKING TIME | SERVING |
|---|---|---|
| 30 mins | 45 mins | 4 |

### INGREDIENTS

1 medium head of cabbage
500g lean ground turkey or chicken
1 cup cauliflower rice
1 small onion, finely chopped
2 garlic cloves, minced
1 medium zucchini, diced
1 medium tomato, diced
1 tsp ground cumin
½ tsp paprika

### DIRECTIONS

1. Prepare the cabbage leaves by boiling the cabbage head until leaves are pliable. Remove and set aside.
2. For the filling, in a skillet, sauté onion and garlic in olive oil until translucent. Add ground turkey/chicken and cook until no longer pink. Stir in zucchini, tomato, cumin, paprika, salt, and pepper. Add cauliflower rice and cook for 5 minutes

1 tbsp olive oil
Fresh parsley for garnish (optional)

3. Assemble cabbage rolls by placing filling in each cabbage leaf and rolling it up.
4. Cook by preheating the oven to 180°C (350°F). Arrange cabbage rolls seam-side down in a baking dish, cover with foil, and bake for 30-35 minutes.

**Nutritional facts /value (per serving)**

| **Cal:** 170 | **Carbs:** 10g | **Protein:** 20g | **Total Fats:** 7g | **Sodium:** 90mg |
|---|---|---|---|---|
| **Pott:** 670mg | **Calcium:** 50mg | **Phos:** 220mg | **Fiber:** 3g | **Sugar:** 6g |

## 10.16 ALLERGY FRIENDLY BUCKWHEAT PANCAKES

| PREPARATION TIME | COOKING TIME | SERVING |
|---|---|---|
| 10 mins | 15 mins | 4 |

**INGREDIENTS**
1 cup buckwheat flour
1.5 cups almond milk
1 egg (or flaxseed egg for egg allergy)
1 tbsp olive oil
1 tsp baking powder
Pinch of salt

**DIRECTIONS**
1. Combine all the ingredients in a bowl until thoroughly mixed.
2. Heat a non-stick skillet over medium heat and ladle in the batter to form pancakes.
3. Cook until bubbles form on the surface, then flip and cook the other side.

**Nutritional facts /value (per serving)**

| **Cal:** 130 | **Carbs:** 22g | **Protein:** 4g | **Total Fats:** 3g | **Sodium:** 190mg |
|---|---|---|---|---|
| **Pott:** 230mg | **Calcium:** 80mg | **Phos:** 0mg | **Fiber:** 4g | **Sugar:** 1g |

## 10.17 ALLERGY FRIENDLY LENTIL SOUP

| PREPARATION TIME | COOKING TIME | SERVING |
|---|---|---|
| 10 mins | 30 mins | 6 |

**INGREDIENTS**
2 cups green lentils, rinsed and drained
1 large onion, chopped
3 garlic cloves, minced
2 carrots, chopped
1 celery stalk, chopped
1 can (400g) diced tomatoes
6 cups vegetable broth
2 tsp ground cumin
1 tsp ground coriander
½ tsp smoked paprika
2 bay leaves

**DIRECTIONS**
1. In a large pot, heat a bit of olive oil over medium heat. Add the onions and garlic, and sauté until golden.
2. Add carrots and celery to the pot and stir for another 5-7 minutes.
3. Stir in the lentils, tomatoes, and spices, mixing well to combine.
4. Pour in the vegetable broth and add bay leaves. Bring the soup to a boil, then reduce the heat and simmer for 25-30 minutes or until the lentils are tender.

Fresh parsley to garnish

5. Remove the bay leaves and adjust the seasoning if necessary.
6. Serve hot, garnished with fresh parsley.

**Nutritional facts /value (per serving)**

| Cal: 210 | Carbs: 36g | Protein: 13g | Total Fats: 1g | Sodium: 300mg |
|---|---|---|---|---|
| Pott: 690mg | Calcium: 60mg | Phos: 180mg | Fiber: 14g | Sugar: 6g |

## 10.18 ALLERGY-FRIENDLY SWEET POTATO AND BLACK BEAN BURGERS

| PREPARATION TIME 20 mins | COOKING TIME 25 mins | SERVING 4 |
|---|---|---|

**INGREDIENTS**

2 large sweet potatoes, peeled and diced
1 can (400g) black beans, drained and rinsed
½ cup gluten-free rolled oats
¼ cup finely chopped red onion
2 cloves garlic, minced
1 tsp ground cumin
½ tsp smoked paprika

2 tbsp olive oil
Gluten-free burger buns or lettuce wraps
Toppings like avocado, dairy-free cheese, lettuce, tomato, and dairy-free mayo

**DIRECTIONS**

1. Steam and Mash Sweet Potatoes: Steam the diced sweet potatoes until soft (about 10-15 minutes). Mash them in a large bowl.
2. Combine Ingredients: Add black beans, rolled oats, red onion, minced garlic, ground cumin, smoked paprika, salt, and pepper to the mashed sweet potatoes. Mix until well combined.
3. Form Patties: Divide the mixture into 4 portions and shape them into burger patties.
4. Cook Patties: Heat olive oil in a skillet over medium heat. Cook the patties for about 4-5 minutes on each side until golden brown.
5. Assemble Burgers: Place the cooked patties on buns or lettuce wraps. Add toppings like avocado, dairy-free cheese, lettuce, tomato, and dairy-free mayo

**Nutritional facts /value (per serving)**

| Cal: 32 | Carbs: 57g | Protein: 11g | Total Fats: 6g | Sodium: 280mg |
|---|---|---|---|---|
| Pott: 600mg | Calcium: 40mg | Phos: 150mg | Fiber: 11g | Sugar: 4g |

## 10.19 ALLERGY-FRIENDLY ROOT VEGETABLE HASH

| PREPARATION TIME | COOKING TIME | SERVING |
|---|---|---|
| 15 mins | 30 mins | 4 |

**INGREDIENTS**

2 cups sweet potatoes, diced
1 cup parsnips, diced
1 cup carrots, diced
2 tbsp olive oil
1 tsp rosemary, finely chopped
1 tsp thyme, finely chopped

**DIRECTIONS**

1. Preheat your oven to 400°F (200°C).
2. In a large mixing bowl, combine the diced sweet potatoes, parsnips, and carrots.
3. Add the olive oil, rosemary, and thyme to the vegetable mixture and stir well to coat.
4. Spread the mixture evenly on a baking tray.
5. Bake for 25-30 minutes or until the vegetables are tender and slightly caramelized.
6. Season with .
7. Serve warm as a side dish or as a main course with a portion of grilled chicken or fish.

**Nutritional facts /value (per serving)**

| Cal: 180 | Carbs: 28g | Protein: 3g | Total Fats: 7g | Sodium: 80mg |
|---|---|---|---|---|
| Pott: 540mg | Calcium: 50mg | Phos: 85mg | Fiber: 6g | Sugar: 7g |

## 10.20 ALLERGY-FRIENDLY STUFFED ACORN SQUASH

| PREPARATION TIME | COOKING TIME | SERVING |
|---|---|---|
| 15 mins | 45 mins | 4 |

**INGREDIENTS**

2 acorn squashes, halved and seeds removed
1 cup cooked quinoa
1 cup finely chopped kale
½ cup finely diced carrots
½ cup finely diced red bell pepper
½ cup chopped walnuts (omit if nut-allergic)
Tw tbsp of olive oil
1 tsp ground cinnamon
½ tsp ground nutmeg

**DIRECTIONS**

1. Preheat your oven to 400°F (200°C).
2. Place the acorn squash halves on a baking tray, cut side up, and drizzle with a tbsp of olive oil. Season with salt and pepper.
3. Roast the squash in the preheated oven for about 30-35 minutes or until tender.
4. Meanwhile, take a bowl, a combine quinoa, chopped kale, diced carrots, and diced red bell pepper.
5. In a skillet, heat the remaining olive oil over medium heat. Add the quinoa mixture and cook for about 7-8 minutes, stirring occasionally.
6. Stir in the cinnamon and nutmeg to the quinoa mixture.
7. Once the squash is ready, remove from the oven and let it cool slightly.

8. Fill each squash half with the quinoa mixture, pressing down gently to pack the filling.
9. Return the filled squash to the oven and bake for an additional 10-15 minutes.

| Nutritional facts /value (per serving) | | | | |
|---|---|---|---|---|
| Cal: 200 | Carbs: 30g | Protein: 6g | Total Fats: 8g | Sodium: 60mg |
| Pott: 600mg | Calcium: 80mg | Phos: 100mg | Fiber: 5g | Sugar: 3g |

# 11. PART IV: THE 30-DAY LIVER REJUVENATION MEAL PLAN

## 11.1 PREPARING FOR SUCCESS: SETTING UP YOUR KITCHEN AND PANTRY

**Essential Kitchen Tools:**

A well-equipped kitchen is essential for preparing liver-friendly meals. Ensure you have the following tools:

- Sharp knives for precise slicing.
- Cutting boards for safe food prep.
- Non-stick cookware for healthier cooking with less oil.
- Measuring cups and spoons to control portion sizes.
- Blender or food processor for making smoothies and purees.

**Pantry Staples:**

Stock your pantry with these fatty liver-friendly staples:

- Whole grains foods like whole-wheat pasta, brown rice, and quinoa.
- Olive oil or avocado oil for cooking.
- Flavor-enhancing herbs and spices without excess saltiness.
- Low-sodium broths & canned vegetables.
- Nuts and seeds for healthy snacking.

**Organizing Your Kitchen:**

A well-organized kitchen can make healthy cooking a breeze:

- Arrange your pantry with liver-friendly items at eye level.
- Keep fresh produce easily accessible in the fridge.
- Label and date pantry items to reduce food waste.
- Use clear containers for easy ingredient identification.

**Food Safety:**

Prioritize food safety to protect your liver:

- Wash fruits and vegetables thoroughly.
- Store raw meat separately from other foods.
- Cook poultry and pork to safe temperatures.
- Refrigerate leftovers promptly to prevent spoilage.

**Meal Planning:**

Plan your meals to support liver health:

- Create a weekly meal plan with liver-friendly recipes.
- Add a diverse selection of vibrant fruits & veggies.
- Incorporate lean/very lean protein sources like fish and tofu.
- Limit processed foods high in saturated fats and sugars.

**Ingredient Substitutions:**

Learn how to make healthier swaps:

- Replace refined grains with whole grains.
- Substitute Greek yogurt for sour cream or mayonnaise.
- Use herbs and spices in place of excessive salt.
- Experiment with alternative sweeteners like honey or stevia.

By setting up your kitchen and pantry with these guidelines in mind, you'll be well-prepared to embark on your journey to manage fatty liver disease through wholesome and nutritious cooking. Properly equipping your kitchen and stocking your pantry with liver-friendly ingredients will make it easier to follow the dietary recommendations and recipes in this cookbook, ultimately supporting your liver health and overall well-being.

## 11.2 WEEK-BY-WEEK BREAKDOWN WITH DAILY MENUS

**Week 1:**

| Days | Breakfast | Snack | Lunch | Snack | Dinner |
|---|---|---|---|---|---|
| Day 1 | Papaya Bowl | Nutty Berry Energy Balls | Spinach And Beet Salad | Apple & Walnut Crunch Mix | Vegetable And Quinoa Casserole |
| Day 2 | Detox Bowl | Good Fat Avocado Dip | Quinoa And Chickpea Salad With Tahini | Seed Crackers | Sweet Potato And Lentil Pie |
| Day 3 | Turmeric And Mango Smoothie | Crispy Zucchini Chips | Kale Salad With Avocado And Lime Dressing | Citrus Fruit Mix | Eggplant And Chickpea Casserole |
| Day 4 | Walnut And Blueberries Bowl | 2 Ingredients Kale Chips | Roasted Vegetable Salad With Balsamic Vinegar | Kiwi And Berry Bliss | Mushroom And Turkey Casserole |
| Day 5 | Carrot And Ginger Smoothie | Vegan Artichoke Spinach Dip | Citrus Avocado Salad With Orange | Tropical Papaya & Pineapple Combo | Brown Rice And Spinach Casserole |
| Day 6 | Beetroot And Berry Smoothie | Delicious Beet Dip | Grilled Chicken And Strawberry Salad | Colorful Fruit Mix | Tuna And Bean Casserole |
| Day 7 | Banana And Walnut Oatmeal | Beetroot Chips | Grilled Chicken And Avocado Wrap | Berry & Melon Medley | Grilled Salmon With Lemon And Dill |

**Week 2:**

| Days | Breakfast | Snack | Lunch | Snack | Dinner |
|------|-----------|-------|-------|-------|--------|
| Day 1 | Apple And Cinnamon Oatmeal | Garlic And Lemon Cashew Dressing | Mediterranean Hummus Wrap | Nutty Berry Energy Balls | Vegetable And Quinoa Casserole |
| Day 2 | Mixed Berries Oatmeal With Chia Seeds | Liver Friendly Seeds Mix | Turkey And Cranberry Sandwich | Seed Crackers | Sweet Potato And Lentil Pie |
| Day 3 | Spinach And Mushroom Oatmeal | Seed And Nut Butter | Roasted Vegetable And Hummus Wrap | Good Fat Avocado Dip | Eggplant And Chickpea Casserole |
| Day 4 | Pumpkin Pie Oatmeal | Chia Seed And Almond Drink | Lettuce And Egg Wrap | Crispy Zucchini Chips | Mushroom And Turkey Casserole |
| Day 5 | Banana Walnut Pancake | Seed Crackers | Smoked Salmon And Cucumber Sandwich | Delicious Beet Dip | Brown Rice And Spinach Casserole |
| Day 6 | Blueberry And Almond Pancakes | Chia Seed And Almond Drink | Quinoa And Roasted Vegetable Bowl | Beetroot Chips | Tuna And Bean Casserole |
| Day 7 | Cinnamon Apple Pancakes | Coconut Chia Pudding | Spinach And Lentil Pilaf | Good Fat Avocado Dip | Grilled Salmon With Lemon And Dill |

**Week 3:**

| Days | Breakfast | Snack | Lunch | Snack | Dinner |
|------|-----------|-------|-------|-------|--------|
| Day 1 | Chia Berry Pancakes | No-Bake Protein Cinnamon Balls | Mediterranean Quinoa Bowl | Carrot & Ginger Soup | Vegetable And Quinoa Casserole |
| Day 2 | Spinach And Mushroom Pancakes | Vegan Seeds Energy Balls | Barley And Chickpea Bowl | Nutty Berry Energy Balls | Sweet Potato And Lentil Pie |
| Day 3 | Pumpkin Spice Waffles | Easy Pecan Bars | Quinoa And Lemon Herb Pilaf | Seed Crackers | Eggplant And Chickpea Casserole |
| Day 4 | Avocado And Spinach Breakfast Salad | Beetroot Chips | Mushroom Pilaf | Coconut Chia Pudding | Mushroom And Turkey Casserole |
| Day 5 | Greek Breakfast Salad | Garlic And Lemon Cashew Dressing | Vegetable And Chicken Soup | Delicious Beet Dip | Brown Rice And Spinach Casserole |
| Day 6 | Quinoa And Berry Salad | Seed And Nut Butter | Vegetable And Lentil Stew | Good Fat Avocado Dip | Tuna And Bean Casserole |
| Day 7 | Soaked Salmon Breakfast Salad | Seed Crackers | White Bean And Spinach Soup | Beetroot Chips | Grilled Salmon With Lemon And Dill |

**Week 4:**

| Days | Breakfast | Snack | Lunch | Snack | Dinner |
|------|-----------|-------|-------|-------|--------|
| **Day 1** | Spinach And Avocado Breakfast Salad | Seed Crackers | Rice And Turkey Soup | Nutty Berry Energy Balls | Vegetable And Quinoa Casserole |
| **Day 2** | Chia Yogurt Salad | Garlic And Lemon Cashew Dressing | Tomato And Lentil Soup | Seed Crackers | Sweet Potato And Lentil Pie |
| **Day 3** | Tofu Breakfast Salad | Seed And Nut Butter | Butternut Squash And Apple Soup | Delicious Beet Dip | Eggplant And Chickpea Casserole |
| **Day 4** | Spinach And Mushroom Scrambled Egg | Coconut Chia Pudding | Chickpea And Spinach Curry | Good Fat Avocado Dip | Mushroom And Turkey Casserole |
| **Day 5** | Greek Yogurt Parfait | Seed Crackers | Sweet Potato And Bean Taco | Beetroot Chips | Brown Rice And Spinach Casserole |
| **Day 6** | Breakfast Quinoa Bowl | No-Bake Protein Cinnamon Balls | Quinoa And Vegetable Stir Fry | Nutty Berry Energy Balls | Tuna And Bean Casserole |
| **Day 7** | Chickpea And Spinach Mix | Garlic And Lemon Cashew Dressing | Lentil And Quinoa Salad | Delicious Beet Dip | Grilled Salmon With Lemon And Dill |

# 11.3   TIPS FOR STAYING ON TRACK: DEALING WITH CRAVINGS AND SOCIAL SITUATIONS

Maintaining a fatty liver-friendly diet is crucial for managing your condition and promoting liver health. However, sticking to a specialized diet can be challenging, especially when faced with cravings and social Situations that often involve less healthy food choices. To help you stay on track and make dietary choices that support your liver, here are some valuable tips for handling cravings and navigating social gatherings:

**Dealing with Cravings:**

- **Understand Your Cravings:** Recognize that cravings are a natural part of life, and they often stem from emotional, physical, or psychological factors. By identifying the root cause of your cravings, you can better address them.

- **Plan Healthy Alternatives:** Keep liver-friendly snacks readily available to satisfy your cravings. For example, prepare a batch of liver-friendly energy balls, keep a bowl of fresh fruit handy, or have a small portion of nuts or seeds when cravings strike.

- **Mindful-Eating:** Cultivate the habit of mindful eating by closely focusing on the flavors, textures, satisfaction that comes from healthy foods. This can help you feel more content and less inclined to indulge in unhealthy options.

- **Stay Hydrated:** Often, thirst is mistaken for hunger. When you feel a craving coming on, drink a glass of water first. Sometimes, proper hydration can help curb your appetite.

- **Portion Control:** If you find it challenging to resist your favourite treats, allow yourself small portions occasionally. Moderation is key, and it can help you avoid feeling deprived.
- **Distract Yourself:** When cravings are strong, try engaging in activities that divert your attention away from food. Take a walk, engage in some reading, or practice a hobby to keep your mind occupied.

**Dealing with Social Situations:**

- **Plan Ahead:** If you're attending a social event or gathering, plan your strategy in advance. Consider eating a small, liver-friendly meal before you go to curb your appetite and reduce the temptation to indulge in unhealthy options.
- **Communicate Your Needs:** Don't hesitate to inform your friends and family about your dietary restrictions and the importance of your liver health. Most people will be understanding and accommodating, offering healthier food options.
- **BYO (Bring Your Own):** If you're unsure about the available food choices, bring a liver-friendly dish to share. This ensures that you have something safe to eat and introduces others to nutritious options.
- **Be Selective:** When at a buffet or potluck, choose liver-friendly dishes like salads, lean proteins, and vegetables. Avoid high-fat, fried, and sugary foods that can exacerbate fatty liver disease.
- **Practice Assertiveness:** It's okay to politely decline food that doesn't align with your dietary needs. Use assertive language to decline without feeling pressured or uncomfortable.
- **Focus on Socializing:** Shift the focus of social gatherings from food to conversation and activities. Engage in meaningful discussions and enjoy the company of friends and family to reduce the emphasis on eating.
- **Have a Support System:** Surround yourself with a support network of friends and family who understand your dietary goals and encourage your efforts to maintain liver health.

Remember that staying on track with your fatty liver-friendly diet is a long-term commitment to your health. Cravings and social situations may present challenges, but with the right strategies and a positive mindset, you can navigate these obstacles and continue making choices that support your liver health. Over time, you'll find that healthy eating becomes a natural and satisfying part of your lifestyle.

# 12. PART V: BEYOND DIET: HOLISTIC APPROACHES TO LIVER HEALTH

## 12.1 THE SYNERGY OF EXERCISE AND DIET FOR LIVER FUNCTION

### 12.1.1 Mindfulness, Meditation, and Liver Health

While dietary choices play a vital role in managing fatty liver disease, it's equally important to address the emotional and psychological aspects of your health. Mindfulness and meditation can be powerful tools in supporting your liver health journey. These practices promote mental well-being, reduce stress, and encourage positive lifestyle changes. Here's how mindfulness and meditation can benefit your liver health:

### 12.1.2 Stress Reduction:

- **The Impact of Stress:** Chronic stress can contribute to inflammation and worsen fatty liver disease. High levels of stress hormones can increase the risk of liver damage.
- **Mindfulness for Stress Reduction:** Practices like deep breathing exercises and meditation, which are part of mindfulness techniques, can effectively reduce stress levels. These practices encourage you staying in the present moment, reduce stress and promoting relaxation.

### 12.1.3 Meditation for Stress Relief:

Regular meditation sessions can improve your ability to handle stress. Meditation techniques, like mindfulness meditation, progressive muscle relaxation, or guided imagery, can calm the mind and reduce the physical and emotional toll of stress.

### 12.1.4 Emotional Eating:

- **Emotional Eating and Fatty Liver Disease:** Emotional eating, often driven by stress, can lead to unhealthy food choices and overeating, which can exacerbate fatty liver disease.
- **Mindful Eating:** Mindfulness encourages you to be aware of your eating habits and emotions. Eat mindfully by noticing when you're hungry and enjoying your food with each bite and recognize emotional triggers that lead to overeating.
- **Meditation for Emotional Balance:** Meditation can improve your emotional awareness and resilience. By meditating regularly, you can cultivate a better connection with food and reduce the tendency to use it as a coping mechanism for stress.

## 14.1 TRACKING YOUR PROGRESS: JOURNALS AND APPS

Monitoring your journey towards improved liver health and managing fatty liver disease is essential for success. Here are some tools, journals, and apps that can help you track your progress and stay on course:

1. **Food Diary:** A simple notebook or dedicated food diary can help you record your daily food intake. Note the types and quantities of food you consume, as well as any symptoms or reactions you experience.

2. **Calorie Tracking App:** There are many smartphone apps available that can help you track your daily calorie intake, macronutrients, and micronutrients. Popular options include MyFitnessPal, Lose It!, and Chronometer.

3. **Physical Activity Tracker:** Wearable fitness trackers like Fitbit or smartphone apps (e.g., Apple Health) can monitor your physical activity, steps taken, and calories burned.

4. **Blood Sugar Monitoring App:** If you have diabetes or prediabetes, apps like Glucose Buddy can help you track blood sugar levels and correlate them with your dietary choices.

5. **Weight Tracking App:** Apps like Weight Watchers or Yazio can help you set and track weight loss goals, monitor your progress, and adjust your plan accordingly.

6. **Medication Reminder Apps:** If you're taking medications or supplements, apps like Medisafe can send you reminders to take them as prescribed.

7. **Symptom Tracker:** Use a symptom tracker app to monitor any changes or improvements in liver-related symptoms such as fatigue, abdominal discomfort, or jaundice.

8. **Fitness Apps:** Apps like MyPlate by Livestrong or MyNetDiary can help you plan and track your exercise routines and progress.

9. **Meal Planning Apps:** Apps like Mealime or Paprika can assist in meal planning, recipe organization, and creating grocery lists.

10. **Water Intake Tracker:** Staying hydrated is crucial for liver health. Use apps like WaterMinder to track your daily water intake.

11. **Sleep Tracking Apps:** Poor sleep can impact liver health. Apps like Sleep Cycle or Fitbit can monitor your sleep patterns and provide insights for improvement.

12. **Mood and Stress Tracking Apps:** Chronic stress can affect liver health. Consider using apps like Moodpath or Daylio to track your mood and identify stressors.

13. **Liver Health Apps:** There are specific apps designed for managing liver health and fatty liver disease. These may include educational resources, symptom tracking, and diet advice.

Select the tools that align with your specific goals and preferences. Remember that tracking your progress not only helps you stay accountable but also allows you to make informed adjustments to your diet and lifestyle for better liver health.

## 12.1.5 Healthy Habits:

- **Consistency and Lifestyle Changes:** Consistently following a fatty liver-friendly diet and making lifestyle changes can be challenging. Mindfulness and meditation can help you stay committed to your health goals.

- **Setting Intentions:** Before meals, take a moment to set an intention for your eating experience. This can be as simple as a reminder to choose foods that support your liver health.

- **Staying Present:** Mindfulness encourages you to be fully present during meals. Avoid distractions like television or smartphones, and focus on the taste, texture, and nourishment of the food you're eating.

## 12.1.6 Building Resilience:

- **Adapting to Challenges:** Living with fatty liver disease can be emotionally taxing. Meditation and mindfulness practices build emotional resilience, helping you adapt to the challenges that come with managing a chronic condition.

- **Mindfulness-Based Stress Reduction (MBSR):** Consider enrolling in a mindfulness-based stress reduction program. MBSR combines mindfulness meditation and awareness techniques to help you cope with stress, pain, and illness.

### 12.1.7 Getting Started with Mindfulness and Meditation:

- **Daily Practice:** Dedicate a few minutes each day to mindfulness or meditation. Begin with brief sessions and extend the duration gradually as you become more at ease.
- **Guided Resources:** Many apps and online resources offer guided mindfulness and meditation exercises. These can provide structure and guidance as you begin your practice.
- **Incorporate Mindfulness into Meals:** Practice mindfulness during meals by focusing on the sensory experience of eating. Chew slowly, savor the flavors, and pay attention to your body's signals for hunger and fullness.
- **Consistency is Key:** Like any habit, consistency is essential for mindfulness and meditation to yield long-term benefits. Stick with it, and over time, you'll notice improvements in your overall well-being and your ability to manage fatty liver disease.

By incorporating mindfulness and meditation into your routine, you can complement your dietary efforts in managing fatty liver disease. These practices promote emotional well-being, reduce stress, and create a more mindful approach to food and lifestyle choices, all of which contribute to better liver health.

## 12.2 IMPORTANCE OF SLEEP IN LIVER REGENERATION:

Adequate sleep has a significant role in liver regeneration process and overall liver health. During deep sleep stages, the body engages in critical repair and renewal activities, and the liver is no exception. The liver carries out numerous vital functions, including detoxification, metabolism, and the synthesis of essential proteins. Sleep is when the liver gets the opportunity to focus on regenerating damaged cells and replacing old ones.

Sleep deprivation, on the other hand, disrupts these essential processes. Chronic sleep insufficiency can lead to an imbalance in hormones related to appetite and metabolism, potentially promoting weight gain and insulin resistance, both of which can exacerbate fatty liver disease.

Furthermore, inadequate sleep increases inflammation within the body, including the liver, which may contribute to liver damage and disease progression. To support liver health, it is crucial to prioritize restorative sleep. Target 7-9 hours of good-quality sleep nightly, establish a steady sleep pattern, craft a calming bedtime ritual, and minimize disturbances to your sleep. By doing so, you can enhance the liver's regenerative capabilities and reduce the risk of liver-related complications, ultimately promoting better overall well-being.

## 12.3 NATURAL SUPPLEMENTS AND HERBS FOR LIVER SUPPORT:

In addition to dietary modifications and a healthy lifestyle, natural supplements and herbs can play a valuable role in supporting liver health. These botanical remedies have been used for centuries in traditional medicine and have gained recognition for their potential to enhance functioning ability of the liver and aid in the management of fatty liver disease. Here are some key natural supplements and herbs to consider:

- **Milk Thistle (Silymarin):** Milk thistle is perhaps one of the most well-known herbs for liver support. Its active component, silymarin, has Properties of being antioxidants and having anti-inflammatory effects that can help shield liver cells from harm. Milk thistle supplements are available in various forms, including capsules and extracts.

- **Turmeric:** Curcumin, the active component found in turmeric, is well-known for its anti-inflammatory and antioxidant attributes. It has the potential to alleviate liver inflammation and promote general liver well-being. Turmeric can be ingested as a culinary spice or as a dietary supplement.

- **Dandelion Root:** Dandelion root is believed to support liver health by promoting bile production, which aids in the digestion and detoxification processes. It can be consumed as a tea or in capsule form.

- **Artichoke:** Artichoke extract contains a wealth of antioxidants and substances that bolster liver performance. It might enhance the digestive process, promote the release of bile, and ease symptoms associated with indigestion

- **Ginger:** Ginger possesses anti-inflammatory and antioxidant properties that can benefit liver health. It may help reduce liver damage caused by a high-fat diet and support liver detoxification pathways. You can incorporate ginger into your diet or consume it as a tea or supplement.

- **Licorice Root:** Licorice root is recognized for its possible liver benefits, including anti-inflammatory and antioxidant effects. It may help protect liver cells and promote healthy liver function. You can enjoy licorice root either by brewing it as a tea or taking it in the form of supplements.

- **Green Tea:** Green tea is rich in antioxidants, particularly catechins, which may protect the liver from oxidative stress and inflammation. Regular consumption of green tea can be a simple way to support liver health.

Before adding any supplements or herbal remedies to your regimen, it's crucial to seek advice from a healthcare expert, particularly if you have underlying medical conditions or are using medications. They can offer recommendations regarding suitable dosages and potential interactions with your current treatments. Furthermore, it's important to keep in mind that natural supplements and herbs should be seen as supplementary measures and not substitutes for a balanced diet and a healthy lifestyle in managing fatty liver disease.

# 13. PART VI: NAVIGATING CHALLENGES AND MISCONCEPTIONS

## 13.1 DEBUNKING COMMON MYTHS ABOUT FATTY LIVER:

Fatty liver disease is a prevalent disorder that impact millions of individuals across the globe, yet it often remains shrouded in misinformation. Let's debunk some common myths surrounding fatty liver disease to provide clarity and promote better understanding:

- **Myth: Fatty Liver Disease Only Affects Heavy Drinkers:** While excessive consumption of alcohol can result in the development of alcoholic fatty liver disease and non-alcoholic fatty liver disease (NAFLD) which is far more common. NAFLD is primarily associated with lifestyle factors such as diet, obesity, and sedentary behaviour.

- **Myth: Fatty Liver Is Harmless:** Fatty liver may start as a benign condition, but it can progress to more severe forms, including Non-alcoholic steatohepatitis (NASH), a condition that can progress to liver fibrosis, cirrhosis, and even liver cancer, underscores the importance of early detection and lifestyle modifications.

- **Myth: Fatty Liver Is Irreversible:** Fatty liver disease is often reversible, especially in its early stages. Making lifestyle adjustments, which include changing your diet, engaging in physical activity, and achieving weight loss, can enhance liver health and diminish fat buildup.

- **Myth: Medications Alone Can Cure Fatty Liver:** While some medications may be prescribed to manage symptoms and underlying conditions, there is no specific medication that universally cures fatty liver disease. Lifestyle changes remain the cornerstone of treatment.

## 13.2 OVERCOMING SETBACKS IN YOUR LIVER HEALTH JOURNEY:

Managing fatty liver disease can be challenging, and setbacks may occur along the way. Here are some strategies to help you stay resilient and focused on your liver health journey:

1. **Seek Support:** Share your experience with either friends, family members, or a support group. Possessing a community of individuals who grasp your situation and provide encouragement can offer significant advantages.

2. **Mindful Eating:** If you slip up or have a setback, don't let it derail your progress. Practice mindful eating, acknowledge the setback, and refocus on making healthy choices.

3. **Regular Monitoring:** Stay in touch with your healthcare provider for regular check-ups and liver function tests. This can help you track your progress and catch any issues early.

4. **Set Realistic Goals:** Be patient with yourself and set achievable goals. Sustainable lifestyle changes often take time, so celebrate small victories along the way.

5. **Stay Informed:** Continue educating yourself about fatty liver disease and the latest research. Knowledge empowers you to make educated choices concerning your well-being.

6. **Professional Guidance:** You might want to think about seeking personalized advice from a registered dietitian or a liver specialist. They can help you develop a tailored nutrition plan and provide expert advice.

It's important to keep in mind that facing challenges is a normal aspect of any health journey. What matters most is your commitment to getting back on track and making choices that support your liver health. With perseverance and a proactive approach, you can overcome obstacles and work toward a healthier, happier life.

## 13.3   THE ROLE OF MEDICATION: WHEN DIET ISN'T ENOUGH

While a healthy diet and lifestyle modifications are foundational in managing fatty liver disease, there are instances where medication becomes a valuable component of treatment. Here, we explore the role of medication when dietary changes alone aren't sufficient to address this condition:

1. **Controlling Underlying Conditions:** For individuals with non-alcoholic fatty liver disease (NAFLD) who have coexisting health conditions like diabetes, high blood pressure, or high cholesterol, medication may be prescribed to manage these conditions effectively. Controlling these underlying conditions can have a positive impact on liver health.

2. **Managing Advanced Stages:** In cases where fatty liver disease has progressed to non-alcoholic steatohepatitis (NASH) or liver fibrosis, medication may be recommended to slow down or halt the progression of liver damage. Medications such as vitamin E, pioglitazone, or obeticholic acid may be prescribed by healthcare professionals.

3. **Weight Loss Medication:** Some individuals with obesity-related fatty liver disease may benefit from weight loss medications under the supervision of a healthcare provider. These medications can help in achieving and maintaining a healthy weight, which is essential for liver health.

4. **Antioxidants and Anti-inflammatories:** Certain medications, such as antioxidants and anti-inflammatory agents, may be prescribed to combat oxidative stress and inflammation in the liver. Vitamin E and omega-3 fatty acids are examples of supplements that have shown promise in clinical studies.

5. **Experimental Therapies:** Ongoing research is exploring various experimental therapies and medications designed specifically for fatty liver disease treatment. Clinical trials may offer access to these innovative treatments for eligible individuals.

6. **Medication for Symptom Management:** Medication may also be prescribed to manage specific symptoms or complications associated with fatty liver disease, such as itching, fatigue, or elevated liver enzymes.

It's crucial to note that medication should always be considered as part of a comprehensive treatment plan under the guidance and supervision of a healthcare provider. The choice of medication, if necessary, will depend on the individual's specific condition, medical history, and response to treatment.

Ultimately, while medication can be a valuable tool in managing fatty liver disease, it should complement, not replace, a healthy lifestyle, including a balanced diet, regular physical activity, and weight management. Combining these approaches offers the best chance of improving liver health and overall well-being for individuals with fatty liver disease.

# 14. PART VII: RESOURCES AND ADDITIONAL TOOLS

## 14.2 SHOPPING LISTS: PICKING QUALITY INGREDIENTS

**Produce:**
- Papayas
- Detox-friendly fruits and vegetables like kale, spinach, cucumber, and lemon
- Berries (blueberries, strawberries, raspberries)
- Carrots
- Ginger
- Beets
- Apples
- Cinnamon
- Spinach
- Mushrooms
- Pumpkin
- Bananas
- Walnuts
- Almonds
- Avocado
- Greek yogurt
- Quinoa
- Salmon
- Tofu
- Chickpeas
- Lentils
- Barley
- Rice
- Tomatoes
- Butternut squash
- Sweet potatoes
- Beans (black beans, white beans)
- Bell peppers
- Eggplant
- Broccoli
- Asparagus
- Snow peas
- Cauliflower
- Kiwi
- Pineapple
- Melons
- Grapes

**Dairy and Dairy Alternatives:**
- Greek yogurt (or dairy-free yogurt)
- Almond milk (or other non-dairy milk)
- Cheese

**Protein:**
- Chicken breast
- Turkey
- Shrimp
- Beef

**Pantry Staples:**
- Oatmeal
- Pancake/waffle mix (or ingredients like flour, baking powder, etc.)
- Quinoa
- Lentils
- Chickpeas
- Brown rice
- Quinoa
- Barley
- Canned beans (black beans, white beans)
- Canned tomatoes
- Broth (chicken, vegetable)
- Olive oil
- Coconut oil
- Spices (turmeric, cinnamon, paprika, etc.)
- Herbs (basil, oregano, etc.)
- Salt and pepper
- Vinegar (balsamic, apple cider, etc.)

- Nuts and seeds (walnuts, chia seeds, pumpkin seeds, etc.)
- Nut and seed butter (peanut butter, almond butter)
- Tea (green tea, herbal tea)
- Canned or dried fruits

**Bakery and Grains:**
- Pancake mix
- Whole-grain bread (if needed for sandwiches or toast)
- Whole-grain pasta

**Freezer Section:**
- Frozen berries (for smoothies)
- Frozen vegetables
- Frozen shrimp or other seafood

**Snacks and Treats:**
- Ingredients for homemade energy balls (dates, nuts, seeds, etc.)
- Granola bars
- Dark chocolate
- Fresh fruit for snacking

**Beverages:**
- Green tea
- Herbal teas
- Almond milk (or other non-dairy milk)
- Water

## 14.3  KITCHEN GADGETS TO SIMPLIFY YOUR COOKING

- Blender or Food Processor
- NutriBullet or Personal Blender
- Slow Cooker
- Instant Pot or Pressure Cooker
- Steamer Basket
- Salad Spinner
- Food Scale
- Measuring Cups and Spoons
- Chef's Knife and Cutting Board
- Mandoline Slicer
- Vegetable Peeler
- Non-Stick Cookware
- Stand Mixer (e.g., KitchenAid)
- Hand Mixer
- Immersion Blender
- Grater
- Mixing Bowls
- Whisk
- Tongs
- Silicone Spatulas
- Wooden Spoons
- Colander
- Can Opener
- Thermometer (for checking meat and liquids)
- Baking Sheets and Pans
- Cooling Racks
- Pastry Brush
- Parchment Paper
- Food Storage Containers
- Garlic Press
- Citrus Juicer
- Coffee Grinder (for grinding seeds and spices)
- Food Thermos (for soups and smoothies on the go)
- Digital Timer
- Kitchen Shears
- Spice Grinder
- Microplane Zester

- Egg Separator
- Rice Cooker
- Toaster or Toaster oven

- Food Dehydrator (for healthy snacks)
- Sous Vide Precision Cooker (for precise cooking)

- Electric Grill or Panini Press
- Herb Scissors
- Vegetable Spiralizer

## 14.4 FURTHER READING: BOOKS AND RESEARCH ON LIVER HEALTH

Expanding your knowledge about liver health through books and research can empower you to make informed choices and better manage fatty liver disease. Here are some recommended books and resources to delve deeper into the topic:

**Books:**

1. **"The Liver Healing Diet" by Michelle Lai and Asha Kasaraneni:** This book provides insights into dietary approaches for liver health and includes recipes designed to support liver function.
2. **"The Liver Cleansing Diet" by Dr. Sandra Cabot:** Dr. Cabot explores dietary strategies for detoxifying and supporting the liver, offering meal plans and recipes.
3. **"Fatty Liver: You Can Reverse It" by Sandra Cabot, M.D., and Thomas Eanelli, M.D.:** A comprehensive guide to understanding and reversing fatty liver disease through diet and lifestyle changes.
4. **"The Liver Rescue" by Anthony William:** This book discusses the role of the liver in overall health and offers insights into healing foods and recipes.
5. **"The Complete Idiot's Guide to the Liver and Liver Diseases" by Dr. Rakesh Gupta:** A straightforward guide to understanding liver health, liver diseases, and lifestyle choices that can impact the liver.
6. **"The Liver Healing Workbook" by Michelle Lai and Asha Kasaraneni:** A companion workbook to "The Liver Healing Diet" that includes meal plans, shopping lists, and journaling prompts.

**Research and Scientific Journals:**

1. **PubMed:** A comprehensive database of scientific research articles, PubMed allows you to search for studies related to liver health, fatty liver disease, and related topics.
2. **Journal of Hepatology:** This respected medical journal publishes research on liver diseases, including fatty liver disease and its management.
3. **Liver International:** Another reputable journal that focuses on liver research, offering insights into the latest developments in the field.
4. **American Journal of Gastroenterology:** Covers a wide range of topics related to gastrointestinal health, including liver issues.
5. **Clinical Gastroenterology and Hepatology:** A journal that publishes clinical studies and research related to liver and gastrointestinal health.

6.  **Hepatology:** The official journal of the American Association for the Study of Liver Diseases, providing in-depth research on liver diseases and treatments.

When exploring scientific journals, you may access articles and research papers related to liver health by visiting your local university library or through online databases available at universities or research institutions.

Remember to consult with healthcare professionals and experts when interpreting research findings and applying them to your specific health needs. Reading books and research can enhance your understanding of liver health and empower you to make informed decisions about your diet and lifestyle.

# ANALYTICAL INDEX

# AFTERWORD

In conclusion, your dedication to liver health is an enduring commitment to your overall vitality. Managing fatty liver disease is a lifelong journey, and with each conscientious decision, you are nurturing a healthier future. Maintain your resolve to lead a balanced lifestyle, consistently schedule check-ups with your healthcare provider, and never hesitate to lean on your support network when necessary. With determination and a deepening understanding of liver health, you possess the ability to safeguard and enhance your liver's well-being throughout your lifetime.

# 15. EXCLUSIVE BONUSES

Download instantly and begin exploring a world of flavors with your exclusive bonus collections - each crafted to perfectly complement your new meal plan. Don't miss out on these delicious additions to your culinary library:

- <u>Grocery List</u>: Optimize your shopping with a detailed list tailored to your meal plan.
- <u>12 Practical Tips</u>: Essential strategies to make your daily cooking simpler and more effective.
- <u>More & Limit</u>: Guidance on what to increase and what to limit in your diet.
- <u>90-Day Meal Plan</u>: Detailed daily plans to help you maintain a healthy and balanced lifestyle.

## SCAN HERE to access your bonuses right away!

Made in the USA
Coppell, TX
14 September 2024

37308197R00063